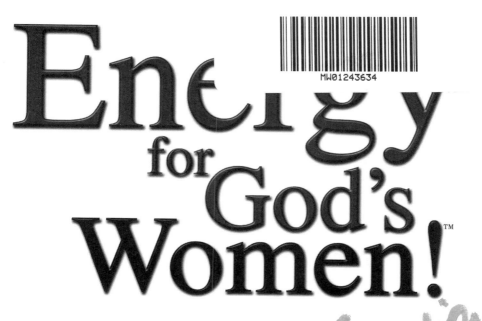

Energy
for God's
Women!™

5 *Steps*

to Restore the Energy,
Joy, and Balance
to Your Life

RUTH GORDON HOWARD

Mission Hills Publishing

ENERGY FOR GOD'S WOMEN!™
Copyright © 2007 Ruth Gordon Howard

Mission Hills Publishing
www.MissionHillsPublishing.com

Howard, Ruth Gordon
Energy for God's Women!™

Library of Congress Control Number: 2006910980

ISBN 13: 978-0-9791489-0-3
ISBN 10: 0-9791489-0-1

Printed in the United States of America

Interior Page Design - Michael Wolff
Cover Design - Jessica Landon
Cover Art "God's Road" – Joan C. Thomson

Scripture quotations marked NASB are taken from the NEW AMERICAN STANDARD BIBLE®, Copyright © 1960,1962,1963,1968,1971,1972,1973,1975,1977,1995 by The Lockman Foundation. Used by permission.

Scripture quotations marked NIV are taken from the HOLY BIBLE, NEW INTERNATIONAL VERSION®. Copyright © 1973, 1978, 1984 International Bible Society. Used by permission of Zondervan. All rights reserved.

Scripture quotations marked NLT are taken from the *Holy Bible, New Living Translation*, Copyright 1996. Used by permission of Tyndale House Publishers, Inc., Wheaton, Illinois 60189. All rights reserved.

Scripture quotations marked MSG are taken from THE MESSAGE. Copyright © Eugene H. Peterson, 1993, 1994, 1995, 1996, 2000, 2001, 2002. Used by permission of NavPress Publishing Group.

Scripture quotations marked NLV are taken from the NEW LIFE Version Bible, Copyright © 1969 Christian Literature International. Christian Literature International (CLI) is a non-profit ministry dedicated to publishing and providing the Word of God. All rights reserved. Used by permission.

When It's All Been Said And Done, Words and Music by James A. Cowan, Copyright © 1999 Integrity's Hosanna! Music/ASCAP, Integrity Media, Inc., 1000 Cody Road, Mobile, AL 36695, All Rights Reserved   International Copyright Secured Used by Permission.

This publication is intended to provide helpful and informative material on the subjects addressed in this publication. It is sold with the understanding that the author and publisher are not engaged in rendering medical, health or psychological, or any other kind of personal services in the book. If the reader requires personal medical, health or other assistance or advice, a competent professional should be consulted. The author and publisher specifically disclaim all responsibility for any liability, loss, or risk, personal or otherwise, that is incurred as a consequence, directly or indirectly of the use and application of any of the contents of this book.

Thanks...

My heartfelt thanks to my two favorite Energy Girls, Tina Mendieta and Dana Mather. Tina, your love for God, faith, and endless energy are a constant joy to me. It's a special blessing to encourage other women with you by my side. Thanks too, for your tireless work on the production of this book. Dana, your loyalty, hard work, faithfulness and friendship helped to build our women's ministry from the ground up. I thank the Lord for you both. You're God's women.

Very special thanks to Barbara Brabec, Patricia Dorazio, Chris Sullivan, Steve and Janie Peklenk, Dave and Anne Gaines, the Sircar family, Jim Powell, Frederick R. Jorgenson, and Charles Cox. Thank you for your gifts of love, friendship, guidance, help, support and prayers.

To my dear, sweet, wonderful husband, Brian—thank you with all my heart for your unconditional support, love, and, most importantly, leading me to Jesus every day. Looking at life through your brilliant, creative eyes is a complete inspiration. You're the love of my life.

This book is dedicated to *you*.

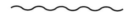

It is my prayer that as you read this book
God will encourage your heart.

Contents

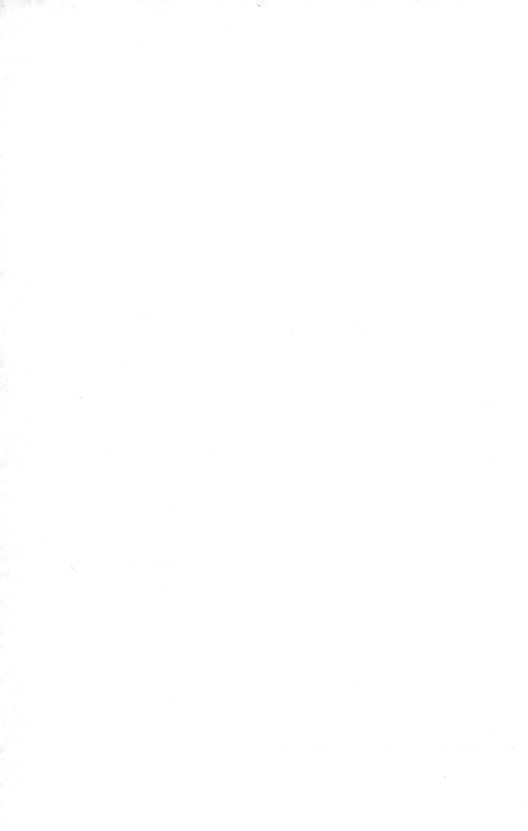

Introduction

My friend...

Are you tired today? Let me assure you, if you feel you are simply surviving instead of really living, you are not alone. Women today are simply over-the-top exhausted.

Would you like to learn how to renew your energy and bring back the balance in your life? Would you like to wake up in the morning with hope and joy? Would you like to have less stress? You *can* have more energy every day.

In my work over the last two decades, I have observed time and time again that it does not matter their age or background or place of work—whether outside the home or in it— women everywhere have the very same complaint: "Help, I'm TIRED!"

As a health professional, I've always tried to share God's principles in a clear, simple way. I'm excited about also sharing my faith in this book, because without the Lord, the true source of all energy and life, there is *no* real help. I believe God has called me to share health information with women just like you.

My mission is to inspire and encourage women to restore the energy, joy, and balance in their lives. I have worked with thousands of women—seeing what worked and what didn't. In my work over the years, one thing is clear—the reasons women are tired are often not physical!

My passion is to help women live healthier lives with joy and energy to spare. Women are not only tired … they are *hurting*. They have been bombarded with the message that they can have it all and do it all, and many have succumbed to the insanity of trying to live that way.

We are physical, emotional, and spiritual beings, and in order to turn things around we need to understand how each of these important elements operates. In my work over the years, I have discovered five key elements that can help provide a way for women to revive their energy and see life in a completely new way.

To begin with, every woman needs to know what her unique and special God-given gifts are, and how to use them. Using your gifts every day will fill you with joy and energize you. I will show you how.

Second, healthy relationships provide support, comfort, hope and, yes, energy when times are tough. Even unhealthy relationships can sometimes be renewed and restored. Steps can be taken to minimize the painful effects of relationship challenges. I will share some simple ways to do this.

Third, women everywhere are overwhelmed by the clutter in their lives. Physical clutter is robbing women of the ability to get things done and is underestimated in its ability to drain away daily energy. I will teach you a simple way to get rid of clutter forever.

Fourth, every woman needs to understand the basics of how to take charge of her physical health. By creating a plan and knowing how to deal with the special health concerns you face as a woman, I can show you how to have more energy immediately.

Finally, women who understand their personal mission and purpose know where God wants them to invest their energy. You don't have time to do it all and, thank goodness, you don't have to. The importance of these five key areas in your life will become clear and, as we address each one and how to deal with it, the reasons you are so tired will become obvious.

Book introductions often let you know that the author is going to say something relevant, helpful, or even life-changing. I want to share something from my heart.

I've devoted my entire career to helping women live healthier lives because absolutely nothing gives me more joy than seeing women live up to their potential, fulfill their dreams, and live lives full of energy. More than anything, I hope this book will give you new insights, help you make beneficial changes in your life, and provide relief from day-to-day exhaustion.

As you read this book, it is my prayer you will begin to experience a sense of renewal. There is hope. There is an answer. If you want more energy, joy, and balance in your life, I have written this book just for you.

Wishing you joy and never-ending energy,

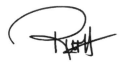

Ruth

As you read this book...

Insights

Look for insights because insight is the key to change and the key to increasing your energy. As you read, take the important step of incorporating new insights into your daily routine. This can literally change your life. Insights are the key to finding hope, a new approach, and a fresh start. I will teach you important principles and you may have heard some of them before. The difference is that sometimes we hear something, and then other times we get an insight and we *really hear* it. Learning, listening, and gaining personal *insight* are the keys. So remember, "Nothing is new under the sun" (Eccles.1:9), but make this the day you use the truth and your insights to turn things around.

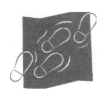

Action Steps

Take action steps. Sometimes we think our good intentions are enough. They're not. Pray and ask God what action steps he wants you to take. My plan will help you. If you have a setback, don't give up. Just get right back on track and keep moving toward your goal. You *will* make progress if you do that, even if some days you feel like you're taking one step forward and two steps back. It's your overall progress that counts. The tortoise didn't just finish the race; she won it by slow, steady determination. Make a commitment to take action steps within 24 hours of gaining an insight, and you will be on the road to success.

Girlfriends to the Rescue

Develop a support network of girlfriends. You can't do it alone. Girlfriends can come to the rescue. A girlfriend and sister in the faith can be an accountability partner. You need someone who will encourage you—and help you make needed changes in your life—to increase your energy. There are countless times we lose perspective. We think things are far worse than they are, and we need someone who can give us a hand and help us keep going— someone who can give us new perspective on a situation. There's always hope. If you know a woman of faith who can be a wise, godly girlfriend, share any insights you gain with her, get her opinion, and stay accountable.

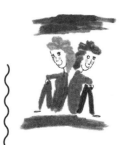

Good News

Pray and ask the Lord for guidance. Remember, no matter what shape you're in now or how tired you are, prayer can deepen your relationship with Jesus, and he is *the* answer. Just focus your heart on him and ask for his help. Simply and humbly.

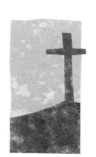

The Lord knows everything about you—all your thoughts, pains, burdens, and fears. He created you to be his unique woman. I don't know the exact challenges you face today, but God knows. I don't know if your heart is broken or full of joy, but God knows. He sees it all. No matter where you've been, what you've done, or what might happen in the future, God loves you in a real and personal way, beyond anything you can imagine. He wants to help you. It's not too late. That's very good news which every woman needs to hear. With God you can experience hope, renewal, and a fresh start.

Join the Energy Girls®!*

Energy Girls® are on a mission to be the best they can be, filled with energy in every season of their lives. Energy Girls® are women who understand the importance of supportive, life-changing relationships with other women. No one can make it alone. Energy Girls® come from every background. They are all ages, shapes, and sizes. What does it take to join us? It starts with a simple commitment to live a healthy lifestyle and a desire to be the best woman you can be, right now, in whatever situation or station of life you find yourself. Look for Energy Girls® *Tips*, *Facts*, and *Questions* as you read this book.

*Dear Men,
A special note to all the men in our lives whom we love, respect and can't live without—our husbands, brothers, relatives and friends. Why do we use the term *girls*? When women call each other *girls*, it's an affectionate term of friendship, fellowship, bonding, and camaraderie. When men call us *girls*, however, we don't take it too kindly. Sorry, that's just one of those "girl things" we hope you'll understand. It's nothing personal, it's just ... girl talk!

Hope and God's Good Plans...

"For I know the plans I have for you,"
declares the LORD, "plans to prosper
you and not to harm you, plans to
give you hope and a future."

Jeremiah 29:11 (NIV)

～～～～

Wonderfully Made ...

I will give thanks to you,
for I am fearfully and
wonderfully made.

Psalm 139:14 (NASB)

~~~~~~~~

Help! I Need Energy

When you woke up this morning, were you refreshed and rested? How much energy did you have? At the start of a brand new day, were you hoping and praying you would have enough energy to take care of everyone and everything, enough energy to *last* until bedtime?

Lack of energy is the number one complaint among working women everywhere, and you must remember *whoever* you are and *wherever* you are—whether at home or in an office—*you are a working woman.*

Most women are exhausted and don't hold out much hope for things to get better. In fact, most women are discouraged about ever getting the extra energy they need—and with that discouragement comes even further exhaustion.

But here is good news. I believe my program will not only give you more energy, but bring joy, hope, and balance back to your life.

Let Me Introduce Hope

Your quality of life is directly related to how exhausted you are mentally, physically, and emotionally. With the program I'm sharing in this book, you will learn five simple steps that will teach you how to have amazing energy. This program will help you awaken and rekindle the hopes and dreams you may have all but given up, because your personal energy level affects every part of your life, including your self-image, your performance, your health, and your relationships.

Invest Your Energy

We must realize that the daily energy we have is a gift. It must be invested wisely and replenished at least as often as it is spent. Then we need to take a long, hard look at ourselves. What are we doing positive that we can build on—and what are we doing negative that we can simply let go? You must be willing to make changes. You must be determined. Your health and well-being depend on it. And since women are the caretakers and nurturers of the world, our families' health and well-being depend on it, too.

The Spiritual Answer

When you give your life *completely* to the Lord, everything changes. All his promises are true for you:

> **The Lord your God has arrived to live among you. He is a mighty savior. He will rejoice over you with great gladness. With his love, he will calm all your fears.**
>
> Zephaniah 3:17a (NLT)

> **As soon as I pray, you answer me; you encourage me by giving me strength.**
>
> Psalm 138:3 (NLT)

Give me happiness, O Lord, for my life depends on you.

Psalm 146:5 (NLT)

"I will take care of you, I made you and will take care of you," says the Lord.

Isaiah 46:4 (NIV)

If you don't have a relationship with Jesus, the one who created you, designed you and made you, you will miss out on the greatest energy source you could possibly have. He can give you true purpose and passion in life, and he is the one who will make it possible for you to not only survive but even *thrive* in the hard times by letting go of the heavy burdens and trusting God to carry them for you. I study the Bible—it's my map and guide for life—and if you're like me at all, when you feel lost you know it helps to have a map. If you read his Word, pray for wisdom and step out in faith. He will bless you.

> **You know me inside and out, you know every bone in my body; you know exactly how I was made, bit by bit, how I was sculpted from nothing into something. Like an open book, you watched me grow from conception to birth; all the stages of my life were spread out before you. The days of my life all prepared before I'd even lived one day.**

Psalm 139:15-16 (MSG)

Without a relationship to the Lord—the true source of energy and joy—we can never be our best or our happiest. Did you know that the word "enthusiasm" literally means "filled with God"? The right spiritual foundation gives us something more powerful than ourselves to look to when all our resources are drained and depleted. How encouraging it is to know with certainty that God loves each of us, no matter who we are and what we may have done in the past. How comforting it is to know that he wants only the best for us and that he is eager to help us attain the goals and dreams he has placed within us—if we will only open our hearts. Are you God's woman? *You can be.*

Energy Emergency

One bright Spring day, Pat was sitting at her kitchen table enjoying a cup of morning coffee. She had just baked some biscuits and was about to take some to her son, Chip, who was in the driveway, working on his new car. Suddenly, Pat heard a loud crash. She rushed out the back door to find Chip pinned under his car.

Energy Girls® Fact!

Pat was only five feet tall and weighed 100 pounds, yet she lifted a car to save her son.

Her only son, Chip—who could barely breathe with the weight of the automobile pushing down on his chest—managed to whisper, "Lift the car, Mom." Pat is only five feet tall and weighs little more than a hundred pounds, but she reached down and lifted the car, saving her son's life.

A few days later they laughed in the hospital about the incident. Chip had a few crushed ribs and Pat had several crushed vertebrae. A friend asked, "Chip, why did you tell your mother to lift the car?" He responded, "I don't know, it was all I could think of to say and, doggone it, she did it. I just call her Supermom now!"

Any mother knows that when her child is in trouble, she truly does have the energy of a Superwoman—at least in the moment of crisis. You may never have to lift a car, but do you have the energy to respond to other emergencies you might encounter?

Do you have energy for your work and all your daily activities? Do you have energy to relax with your family and friends and enjoy fun activities? Every aspect of life requires energy.

Your Stress Response

How did tiny little Pat lift that heavy car? Where did she get the energy? Surely a mother's love energized Pat and enabled her to save her son. Thank God for the mothers of the world who always rise to the occasion.

Physiological factors also contributed to Pat's ability to lift the car. Her body sprang into action voluntarily, the same way your body would if faced with a similar emergency. The same physiological response Pat had occurs inside of you whenever you are under too much stress. God created your body miraculously. Your body's reaction to stress is designed by God to protect you and help you in an emergency, but today we are under constant stress.

One factor working here is known as the "stress response" or the "flight or fight" response. Pat's brain, specifically the hypothalamus, automatically sent her pituitary gland a signal, which in turn sent another signal to the adrenals which lie on top of the kidneys. Then *whoosh*, the release of hormones, better known as the "adrenaline rush," occurred. Pat suddenly became Superwoman with a burst of energy enabling her to do the impossible. If you're a woman of faith, you know God gave her that strength. You have the exact same response in your body every time you are under stress. Your body doesn't differentiate between the kinds of stressful emergencies you

Energy Girls® Fact!

If you're a woman under constant stress and pressure, your body can't handle that kind of stress indefinitely. Sooner or later, it will affect your health—mentally, emotionally, or physically.

are facing; it's a voluntary response from your body, and you're not controlling it. The problem today is, if you're a woman under constant stress and pressure, your body can't handle that kind of stress *indefinitely*. Sooner or later something has to give. For most women, that means their health, their peace, their ability to cope, or their joy. An accumulation of stress from the small "energy enemies" you face *all day long* can end up being serious enough to affect your health by increasing your risk for heart disease, depression, digestive problems, obesity, and insomnia. What kind of energy enemies do you face all day long?

❏ *Conflicts with loved ones*
❏ *Draining relationships*
❏ *Hectic, fast pace—every day*
❏ *Racing against deadlines*
❏ *Working in the home and outside the home*
❏ *Financial problems*
❏ *Too much clutter*
❏ *No time to rest and relax*
❏ *Too many things to do*

Your Personal Energy Enemies

You have *general* energy enemies, but you also have *personal* energy enemies. You respond uniquely and personally to the stress you encounter. You may have different signs and symptoms than another woman, but stress will always rob you both of needed energy. When you are under stress, do you experience any of the following signs and symptoms?

❏ *Overeating*
❏ *Undereating*
❏ *Constant weight gain and weight loss*
❏ *Fatigue*

- ❏ *Headaches*
- ❏ *Back, shoulder, or neck pain*
- ❏ *Nail-biting*
- ❏ *Stomach problems*
- ❏ *Feeling helpless or hopeless*
- ❏ *Guilt that won't go away*
- ❏ *Irritability*
- ❏ *Shortness of breath*
- ❏ *Cold, clammy hands*
- ❏ *Teeth-grinding or jaw-clenching*
- ❏ *Rashes*
- ❏ *Insomnia*
- ❏ *High blood pressure*

If you know how your body responds to stress when your first "stress signals" appear, you can take action. That's the time to do something about it, before you lose additional time, and it takes its toll on your health and energy. Create a plan, with this book as your guide, to control all the *Personal Energy Enemies* that you can. Sometimes you can have *Personal Energy Enemies* that you can't control, but they can be used to make you stronger and even teach you important life lessons.

An important stress principle you must know is that change *always* equals stress. Another energy enemy is too many changes. Most of us live with so much stress and change, we are used to it. For us, it feels normal. You may not remember a time when you didn't feel rushed, hurried, and overwhelmed.

Energy Girls® Tip

Know your personal energy enemies. Learn your personal stress response and take action before stress takes its toll on your health.

The Stress Scale

One of the first attempts to measure stress levels was in 1967, with the Holmes-Rahe Scale. Thomas H. Holmes, MD and Richard H. Rahe, MD, at the University of Washington School of Medicine, created a stress scale based on life-changing events. The scale rated each event and gave them points. Depending on how many points one totaled over a twelve-month span, the likelihood of a health problem, accident, or injury increased. The very highest points were given to major, traumatic life events such as the death of a spouse or a divorce.

A simple way to explain the concept is like this: Have you ever been very busy, perhaps with several life-changing events occurring all at once (you got a new job, had a change in a relationship, a new baby was born, your in-laws came to visit, etc.), when all of a sudden, *wham!* —your immune system gave out and you became ill with a cold, the flu, or some other ailment? It's the same principle. It was that "one more thing"—that very last change—that tipped the scale, and your body just couldn't handle it.

Balance is the Key

Your body tries to maintain "homeostasis" involuntarily. That's your God-given ability to maintain physiological balance, and it's difficult to do with constant change. Just like when you're trying to carry too many grocery bags at one time that you can't balance, one finally drops or breaks. Trying to cope with too many changes at one time can cause illness, rob you of joy or peace, and set you up for exhaustion. Even positive changes, like going on vacation, can rob you of energy because you have to adapt to changes in your routine.

Whenever we have to adapt to change, it takes mental, emotional, and physical resources. You need just the right amount of change to create a life filled with the balance you were meant to have, one that will allow you to give yourself to the things that really count. It's a tension that creates joy and fulfillment.

It's the perfect tension in stringed instruments that creates beautiful music. My husband plays the guitar. When he changes the strings on his instrument, before they're tightened, no music is heard. When he tightens the strings too much, they can actually break. It's only when he tightens the strings just right that beautiful music can be heard and nothing is out of tune. You need just the right amount of change and tension in your life too.

Control What You Can

If you can, try to control the changes in your life. Obviously, there are things you can control and things you can't. If you know, for example, you will be traveling and that's stressful for you, always have the same breakfast on the road that you have at home. That's one less change. If you have to move or change jobs, try to keep everything else in your daily routine the *exact same* during those big life-changing events.

Too Many Options

Too many options can also do the same thing. We certainly have more options than ever before. Consider these facts:

- When a woman goes grocery shopping at a typical supermarket, she's faced with more than 10,000 choices of what to buy.

- Moms make most of the decisions for their kids' activities, and today children can choose between an abundance of optional activities they might go to: music, swim lessons, soccer, dance lessons, art, ice skating or gymnastics. Of course, mom's driving.
- In a few short decades we've gone from three TV networks to the option of choosing between 155+ channels.
- With iTunes and music on our phones, we also have the option of choosing between two million songs.
- We now shop 24/7 in stores, on TV, and online, with the ability to choose between buying millions of items and thousands of brands.
- Amazon.com alone provides us with a multimillion-title catalog.
- Women can even have personal jeans designed and created online, made to order and shipped to their door. We can choose every detail with a myriad of options, down to the thread color we want and style of zipper.

Does any woman need this many options?

Options and choices can be a good thing. We are the most blessed women on the planet and in all of history. In America women have a quality of life that is unequaled anywhere in the world. But the reality is that choices and options take time and energy to deal with, and sometimes simpler really is better. When was the last time you were able to take a walk just to relax, not for exercise, but simply to enjoy God's creation? When was the last time you read a book, just for inspiration and pleasure?

I always encourage women to pick a night and have a "low-tech" evening by turning off the TV, the cell phones, the computer, *everything*—then spending time doing one simple thing they wouldn't normally do with those things on. I urge you to carve out an evening just to spend quality time with your family and friends. If you do, you will begin to feel renewed and refreshed.

Don't Panic

When women start to simplify their lives, sometimes they panic. They are so used to being in the busy mode, it all seems strange and unfamiliar. There does seem to be a kind of adrenaline high that comes with being constantly pressured and busy. But at what cost? Women's bodies, minds, and spirits are made to respond to good ol' fashioned things like sun, flowers, fresh air, conversations with live people, good food, and reflective moments.

> *You will keep in perfect peace all who trust in you, whose thoughts are fixed on you!*
>
> Isaiah 26:3 (MSG)

Tend and Befriend

For decades, health professionals have talked about the stress response and what happens to our bodies during this process. Now, the latest research also shows that women respond in a very unique way to stress. Their special hormones play a role. It's called "tend and befriend." The bottom line is that the special hormones women have, specifically *oxytocin,* cause women to reach out to one another and develop friendships when they are under stress— something men don't do.

Energy Girls® Tip

Try to simplify your life. If you're a woman who is busy all the time, it may feel strange and unfamiliar at first. Take one step at a time and make small changes. Small changes can add up to a changed life.

A unique study at the University of California showed that while the "tend and befriend" response is elicited by oxytocin, other factors help maintain tending and befriending, too, such as women's natural ability to socialize and seek out relationships.

These new studies prove the obvious to even the casual observer: women respond differently than men. Your body is created and designed to do amazing things without your even thinking about it. One of those things is to reach out to your girlfriends for help and support when you're having an energy crisis.

Stress Management is Crucial

Since your body cannot distinguish between lifting a car, fighting with your spouse, or being stuck in a traffic jam, you must be determined to change patterns in your life that are producing stress, with its obvious energy drain. Remember, your body responds voluntarily, expending incredible energy—unless you decide to do something about it. Because your energy is not limitless, the same adrenaline rush that may save you in an emergency can eventually cause exhaustion and a complete meltdown, if repeated often enough.

So, What's a Girl to Do?

There are specific things we can do to decrease stress in our lives and restore the energy we so desperately need. We need to examine what can help us and, after thoughtful consideration of our own *personal* challenges and struggles, decide what the best course of action is to change our situation and turn it around.

First, You Need a Plan

Over the last two decades of helping women restore their energy, I have learned that most women struggle and finally give in to the over-the-top, dizzying pace of our current culture. But if you give in, you will never have the energy, peace, and joy you want. That is why you need a plan. *You need to do things God's way.*

> **The Lord will work out his plans for my life.**
>
> Psalm 138:8 (NLT)

> **The Lord says, "I will guide you along the best pathway for your life. I will advise you and watch over you."**
>
> Psalm 32:8 (NLT)

> **You chart the path ahead of me and tell me where to stop and rest. Every moment you know where I am.**
>
> Psalm 139:3 (NLT)

As you pray about God's plan, ask him to help you live out his purposes for your life. If you understand God's plan and purposes, you will be better equipped to handle any trials and problems that come your way. You can also be confident in the knowledge that God is with you, and you'll experience the joy of knowing you're doing what he's called you to do.

We live in a world that often seems like it has gone crazy with impossible demands and expectations. It's the spiritual foundation we have, as women of faith, that will give us the strength and, yes, energy to do what needs to be done.

As we take this journey together, I want you to consider the following key elements in my five-step plan.

Five Steps to Incredible Energy

Step 1. Your Amazing Gifts

Gifts: Whoever you are, you have been given important gifts, talents, and abilities by God. It's essential that you learn to identify your gifts, learn how to trust and appreciate your gifts, and learn how to incorporate those gifts into your daily activities. Using your unique God-given gifts will add energy, joy, and purpose back in to your life.

Step 2. Relationship SOS

Relationships: Women have many relationship roles. Since we are relationship-oriented, we need to especially ask for God's help to be women of faith, in all the important roles he gives us. When we have difficulty dealing with our emotional ties, it affects every other part of our lives. We will explore simple ways to diminish the impact that stressful relationships can have on you.

Step 3. Declutter Your Life

Declutter: Women need a place where they can rest and find peace. Clutter is robbing women of energy. Physical clutter includes the piles of stuff in closets, offices, kitchen cupboards, and even the clutter in your car. It's draining to live with clutter day in and day out. You need to examine the impact clutter has on your life and learn three simple steps to rid yourself of clutter forever.

Step 4. Your Body's Best Friend

Physical: Your physical well-being is an important element in your having enough energy. Study after study documents that a health-related fitness program and choosing the right things to eat have a profound effect not only on your energy level and sense of well-being, but on reducing your risks for many diseases too. It will improve your health. You will learn the hows and whys of putting the right kind of physical activity back in your life and how to nourish your body so you can have more energy immediately.

Step 5. Your Magnificent Mission

Mission: You need to know God's mission and purpose for your life. Nothing is more important. Once you understand your mission, as God's woman you will find that your time and efforts are more easily dedicated to your highest priorities and purpose. When we get too busy and we're tired, it's easy to lose sight of the one thing that really counts. You will gain a new vision for how to fulfill your true calling.

ENERGY GIRLS® ASSIGNMENT

So, Energy Girl, here is your first assignment: Since insight is the key to change, take the following *Energy Girls® Quick Assessment* which is based on my simple 5-step plan. Then use the *insights* you gain to decide what changes you need to make. Continue to use this assessment until you know you will *never* be tired again!

Energy Girls® Quick Assessment

Energy Girls® Quick Assessment

Even if you think you do not have enough energy now—you *can* increase your *Energy Friends* and decrease your *Energy Enemies.* It's easy and starts with an assessment of your current strengths and weaknesses. Assess your current energy strengths and weaknesses by checking ☑ Yes, Usually or No.

I can clearly explain my priorities and mission to others.

Yes ❑   Usually ❑   No ❑

I can say no when asked to do tasks that are clearly not part of my priorities.

Yes ❑   Usually ❑   No ❑

I can delegate tasks or ask for help when needed.

Yes ❑   Usually ❑   No ❑

I have supportive friends who help me deal **positively** with stress in my life.

Yes ❑   Usually ❑   No ❑

I know what I am good at and use my God-given skills and abilities on a regular basis.

Yes ❑   Usually ❑   No ❑

I do not harbor feelings of anger, resentment or bitterness.

Yes ❑   Usually ❑   No ❑

My home and workspace are organized and I can find things easily.

Yes ❏   Usually ❏   No ❏

I have a "space" I can retreat to when needed that is peaceful, restful and beautiful.

Yes ❏   Usually ❏   No ❏

I know when I feel physical signs of stress and do something positive about it.

Yes ❏   Usually ❏   No ❏

I am active during the day and walk whenever possible.

Yes ❏   Usually ❏   No ❏

I engage in some kind of physical activity that I enjoy on a regular basis.

Yes ❏   Usually ❏   No ❏

I stretch and strengthen my major muscle groups on a regular basis.

Yes ❏   Usually ❏   No ❏

I try to eat whole grain products, fruits and vegetables regularly.

Yes ❏   Usually ❏   No ❏

I limit my intake of fats, sugars, caffeine and "junk foods."

Yes ❏   Usually ❏   No ❏

"Yes" answers are your *Energy Friends*. "Usually" answers are your *Energy Acquaintances*. "No" answers are your *Energy Enemies*. Your goal is to increase your *Energy Friends*.

Look over your answers. Look at your No's first. Don't be afraid of facing the truth about your current situation. Next, look at your Usually's and then your Yes's. Give yourself 1 point for every Yes.

My score _____

Score: (Yes) Energy Friends

12-14 Energy Friends
Congratulations! You're making all the right energy choices and now you can help others.

9-11 Energy Friends
Don't rest on your laurels. You're almost at the top.

5-8 Energy Friends
You have lots of great habits. You can easily build on them to create more energy.

2-4 Energy Friends
You may not have much energy now but there's hope. Start to make 1 or 2 simple changes today.

0-1 Energy Friends
You need to take a long, hard look at your lifestyle choices. You can do it. There's nowhere to go but *up*.

Energy for God's Women

Energy Girls® Questions

Base your answers to the following questions on the *Energy Girls® Quick Assessment* you just took.

- In a few words, what were your No answers?

- What were your Usually answers?

- Did you have any Yes answers? What are they? Those are your strengths.

Where are you now? Answer the following questions on a scale of 1 to 10 (10 being the best, strongest or greatest, and 1 being the worst, weakest or least).

- How easily can you identify your gifts, talents, skills, and abilities? _____

- Are most of your relationships life-giving, positive and healthy? _____

- Is your workspace and living space free from clutter, and do you feel peaceful in your surroundings? _____

- Are you controlling all the things that you can to improve your sense of physical well-being? _____

- Do you understand your mission? Do you understand your priorities, and do you spend most of your time on them? _____

What insight did you gain from answering the above questions?

What are your strengths and what are your weaknesses?

What area would you *like* to work on first to improve your energy level?

- ❑ Gifts
- ❑ Relationships
- ❑ Clutter
- ❑ My body
- ❑ Mission

What is one *specific* action step you can take to do that?

The First Action Step I Can Take _____

Step 1: Your Amazing Gifts

God has given each of you a gift. Use it to help each other. This will show God's loving favor.

1 Peter 4:10 (NLV)

*H*ave you ever felt exhausted but then, unexpectedly, someone asked you to do something you had a natural passion and love to do? All of a sudden you felt a burst of energy that seemed to come from deep within. You can take on tasks with enthusiasm and joy when you're asked to do something that utilizes your natural God-given talents.

You have amazing gifts. I don't care where you are or what you are doing as you read this—whether you are in an office, home with a new baby, running a business, or sitting in the Laundromat. I am here to tell *you* that you have wonderful skills and abilities. God does not leave anyone out. You are unique. One of a kind. No one has your exact combination of talents, life experience, and perspective. The God who created the sun, moon, stars, and galaxies also made you, according to his exact specifications. He gave you *all* your abilities and he wants to show you how to use them.

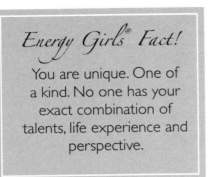

Energy Girls® Fact!

You are unique. One of a kind. No one has your exact combination of talents, life experience and perspective.

Do you have a keen understanding of the wonderful ways you can serve God day to day? If not, it may be because you have not opened your God-given gifts. Once you open them, the exciting journey begins, to find ways to use your gifts the way God intended. The most important key in this venture is to remember that your gifts are given to you *to help others*. And you can be assured the Lord wants you to use your gifts because that's why he gave them to you. When you use the gifts God gave you, it's *energizing*.

Open Your Gifts

Imagine that you're home relaxing when, all of a sudden, you hear a knock on the door. You peer out the window and see an

Energy Girls® Tip

When you use the gifts God gave you, it's energizing.

entourage of people with colorful balloons and a large white van parked out front with a sign that says, "Gift Delivery!" You open the door and are handed a beautifully wrapped package with *your* name emblazoned in gold letters on the box. You are told the gift is from

someone who loves you very much, a secret admirer. It's obvious this is no ordinary gift. Would you say a polite, perfunctory thank-you, take the package, and then walk right back into your house, place the package behind the sofa, and *never touch it again?*

Surely not. When you are given a gift from someone who loves you, it's up to you to *open the gift and use it*.

Energy for God's Wome

Amazing Gifts - Quick Points

1. Ask God to show you what gifts he has given you.
2. God wants you to use your gifts for his purposes.
3. God wants you to give your gifts away.
4. Using your God-given gifts is *energizing!*

~~~~~~~

You've Been Given a Spiritual Gift

The scriptures are clear that all believers have been given a *spiritual* gift. What could be more exciting than to realize that the God who created you from "nothing into something"—the one who is intimately acquainted with all your ways and knows your every thought and desire—also planned on giving you a spiritual gift that would be not only energizing, but just perfect for you to use as you serve him.

When I was a young woman, I gave my life to Christ. From that moment on, I spent time at church learning everything I could. I loved hanging out with the family of God. I couldn't get enough of it. I was the first one at church and the last one to leave. I volunteered for everything from scrubbing floors and cleaning windows to making coffee for Bible study.

One day as I was serving coffee, a friend walked into the church kitchen and it was obvious by his demeanor that he was discouraged. As I poured him a cup, he began to speak about his current depressing circumstances. I listened and started to feel a deep, compelling need to speak up and say something. I had a strong, overwhelming desire to *encourage* him. I simply had to say the words that were very clearly in my heart and mind. Since

I was not raised in the Christian faith, I certainly didn't know the lingo used in most churches, but after I shared what I hoped would help him, he smiled broadly and hollered as he walked out the door, "Why, that sounds just like the word of the Lord! I'm encouraged!" I had definitely never heard anyone say something like that to me before. All I knew was I felt compelled to speak. I had to say what was on my heart, and I thought, "Lord, I'm not sure what just happened here, but I think you were pleased with what I did." I was overjoyed with the sense that God had used me to help someone in a new way.

It wasn't until much later that I learned there was a spiritual gifts test that I could take and that God had been given me the gift of "encouragement" and "exhortation" because he wanted me to use those gifts to help others. Sometimes I get to use that gift in simple ways, like the very first time I was able to encourage and exhort a friend in Christian fellowship as I served coffee. Sometimes I get to use that gift when I'm speaking to many people. It doesn't matter to me, as long as God uses me. No matter how tiring a day might be, I am thrilled and energized if I can encourage anyone, in any way. It's something very deep that God has put in my heart.

What Spiritual Gifts Has God Given You?

One of my girlfriends has the gift of *hospitality* and she is always ready to invite others to her house. It's effortless for her. While she has a flair for making others feel comfortable in her own home, other women I know are "stressed out" at the thought of having company over all the time.

Another girlfriend of mine has the gift of *intercession*. She feels compelled to pray for others. She is passionate about it. It is a serious, spiritual undertaking, but she is always ready to intercede for others and she says this energizes her.

Another girlfriend has the gift of *mercy*. I've never known anyone as compassionate; she is sympathetic and empathic to an amazing degree. How about the gift of *helps*? I have several friends whose great joy it is to simply help others, whenever and wherever they can. No task is too large or too small for them if they can assist.

Do you have the gift of being able to organize large groups that accomplish difficult tasks? I have several girlfriends with the gift of *administration*. Those who don't have the gift are not going to find that task energizing at all. They would be overwhelmed. I also have many friends who are teachers. And who among us has been blessed enough to have our lives changed by a special teacher?

Energy Girls® Fact!
Learning what your spiritual gifts are and how God wants you to use them is a process.

The gift of *teaching* is the very special ability to understand and clearly explain why things are true. We all have different gifts, yet we all need each other.

If you know what spiritual gift God has given you, how are you helping others with your gift? If you have been too busy to even think about it, ask yourself how you could begin *now*, even in a small way, using your spiritual gift?

If you don't know what your spiritual gifts are—and you can have more than one—what steps can you begin to take so you can learn what gifts the Lord has placed within you?

Learning what your spiritual gifts are and how God wants you to use them is a process. It must be built on your relationship with Jesus and the call he has placed on your life. Hopefully, over time, you will grow in your knowledge about what special spiritual gifts you have. It's important to take a spiritual gifts test if you can, but remember, tests are only that—tests. Sometimes they can give you powerful insights and you will feel that ring of truth inside which says, "Yes, I know I have that gift!" But sometimes they can be less than accurate so, when in doubt, pray and ask the people who know you best what they think, then trust what God has placed in your own heart. Then step out in faith, start serving somewhere, and see what the Lord does.

Once you know what your gifts are, you have a responsibility to use them, and you are also accountable to the Lord for what you do with them. When you are using your God-given gifts in the way that pleases God, you will find more energy than you ever thought possible. You might be physically fatigued, but you will also have a deep sense of fulfillment and the very best thing of all—the feeling that you're doing what you were meant to do.

> **Energy Girls® Fact!**
>
> All good gifts come from God. We've been given many gifts that can help restore the energy in our lives—activities that can be refreshing and restful.

Gifts, Gifts and More Gifts!

All good gifts come from God. We've been given many gifts that can help restore the energy in our lives—activities that can be refreshing and restful. Most women today are so busy, they are going from task to task in a blur. Although our lives are filled with more high-tech gadgets than ever before, supposedly to make things simpler and easier, I would like to report that I have never seen so many women burned out, stressed out, and ready to go take a nap.

In the day-to-day frenzy of activity, just trying to keep up with the "to dos" of life has become a stressful challenge. But in case you've forgotten, life is about more than tasks and busyness.

As a woman, you may start to feel like your entire life is problems, troubles, scheduling, and tasks. It's not. Sometimes women focus on meeting everyone else's needs to the point where they become depressed or break down. That's not healthy, and it leaves you with nothing to give to others. How do you add some of those other special gifts back in your life?

There is a wholesome, God-given way to become energized by exploring the things you're naturally passionate about doing. The things you're naturally gifted to do. Even if you're only able to add the things you love back into your life in a very small way, it's a start—and it will give you added energy to meet the needs of others. Do you feel energized by any of the following activities or topics?

❑ Cooking	❑ Fitness	❑ Writing
❑ Painting	❑ Knitting	❑ Nature
❑ Photography	❑ Sewing	❑ Animals
❑ Dancing	❑ Reading	❑ Gardening
❑ Singing	❑ Teaching	❑ Speaking
❑ Music	❑ Crafting	❑ Creating—anything!

If any of the above activities excite you or energize you, maybe it's because you're gifted in that area.

Three Important Questions

For me, there is nothing more exciting than getting to know a new friend and finding out what wonderful gifts she has. Over the years I have had the special opportunity to work with thousands of women, and I have learned that there is an astounding variety in women's talents. I fancy myself something of a treasure hunter now, finding it endlessly fascinating to look for gifts in everyone

I meet. And, do you know, I have yet to come across a single woman who was not gifted in a manner that had the potential to set her apart in a significant way.

No matter what outward impressions may suggest, there is distinct and valuable treasure within each of us, just waiting to be discovered. God is the source of all our hidden talents. He is the source of everything good in our lives.

Every good thing given and every perfect gift is from above, coming down from the Father of lights, with whom there is no variation or shifting shadow.

James 1:17 (NASB)

Another simple way to start exploring and learning what your natural gifts and talents are is by asking yourself three important questions.

1. What do you love to do so much that you lose track of time?

Have you ever found yourself involved in something you loved to do so much that you lost all track of time? What are you passionate about? Your heart and passion are always tied to your gifts.

Do you know what your gifts, skills, talents and abilities are in a broader sense—and do you use them regularly? All good gifts come from God…your abilities, your skills, even your personality type. What excites you, motivates you, or inspires you to take action?

Much has been written about how highly-successful, gifted people found the one thing in life they were passionate about—then just did it. From Bill Gates to Oprah, they all say the same thing: They were passionate about their work when they started, and they still feel that way today. They claim that was the key to their success.

I believe that when we give our lives completely to Christ, he can redeem all our natural interests and passions—all the things that make us uniquely who we are—and use them in a special way for his purposes. We have a choice to let him to do that. We have free will.

From the time I was a little girl, I liked to gather the neighborhood girls together and organize everyone into a group. I remember getting the girls in a circle and then standing up and speaking to them. My father was my hero and the greatest Dad any girl could ask for. He was also a successful TV broadcaster and talk show host. I always watched him closely and probably tried to copy him, but I felt I was doing what

> *Energy Girls® Question*
>
> What do you love to do so much that you lose track of time?

came naturally to me. I believe today that God chose him to be my Dad—that it was in God's sovereign plan—the Lord knew I would have that experience.

When I speak to women's groups today, I love to encourage them. I want to help them discover *their* gifts. That's my passion. I'm very excited to see the light bulbs go on for women and see them energized. I actually enjoy it so much that I lose track of time when I'm doing it, which is why I'm very careful to always wear my watch.

At a conference where I was speaking, I asked the women in the audience this question to further demonstrate a point: "Who here likes to work with numbers?" Now I have never liked dealing with numbers. It's not my gift. I'm grateful for accountants. I am amazed by people who are passionate about working with numbers, and I respect them greatly.

I wasn't surprised when a woman in the back of the room shot her hand up immediately and said, "Yes, I do, I love to work with numbers!" When I asked her if she had always felt that way, she answered, "Yes, always."

Then I asked her if she actually lost track of time when she worked with numbers, and she said, "Oh definitely, I like it that much." Furthermore, she said all of her friends generally wanted her help with different financial and budget questions, and, because she is an accountant, she loves to help people with those problems. In fact, she said that, even when she's tired, if she is asked to help someone with a "numbers" problem she becomes *energized*.

And then I asked her if she could sum up her feelings about numbers for us, especially those of us who may be intimidated by her special skill. With a big smile on her face, she said, "Yes, numbers are my friends." That woman had found her *gift!*

Through the years, the topic of "gifts" has been one of my favorite subjects. Women always seem to love the topic but are usually too tired or too busy to think about it with their overwhelming, day-to-day responsibilities. But if you're tired and asked to do something you love to do, you *will* have the energy to do it. Can you think of something like that in your own life? That's a gift from God.

Even if you're very busy and don't think you have the time now, could you carve out time to rediscover some of those things?

Remember, if you're more energized you can get more done in less time and you will also have more energy to give your family and friends.

2. What do you do easily and effortlessly?

You will surely lose track of time when you're passionate about what you are doing. You will also discover that your true gifts and talents come easily and almost effortlessly to you.

If something comes easily and almost effortlessly for you, I'll bet you're good at it. You might need to develop your potential to do your best in that area, but I believe it will be a helpful puzzle piece to solve the question of how you're gifted. If something is easy and effortless for you, it also energizes you with a feeling of accomplishment.

When you were little, what did you love to do? Do you remember? Sometimes even at a young age, people are so gifted it's breathtaking. Their gifts are obvious to the world, like the most famous child prodigy, Mozart. He wrote his first symphony when he was eight years old. The gifted singer, Celine Dion, was born the youngest of fourteen children in a musical family of very modest means. She started singing as a toddler. At the age of five, her brothers and sisters would put her on top of the kitchen table and she would sing to all of them with a spoon in her hand, pretending it was a microphone. For some people it's very obvious what they should be doing from an early age. However, most of us will need to dig a little deeper to answer this simple question: What seems natural for us—as though we were born to do it?

When we spend all day doing things we are not wired to do, things that don't come easily and naturally for us, it's draining and exhausting. If something is very easy for us, sometimes it's easy to overlook it or to think it's unimportant—but it may be a gift God wants us to use more often.

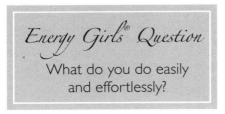

Some of you may be blessed enough to be doing exactly what you're gifted to do every day. If you're not, and the situation is not going to be change anytime soon, commit to putting some of your personal energizers back in your life in small ways—doing the things that are easy and effortless for you.

3. What do others compliment you on?

My husband is an incredibly gifted musician and artist, but others recognized his talents before he did. He started receiving compliments on the songs he wrote as a young adult. It was only after all the compliments that he began to understand his true calling. He is a humble, quiet man, and without others recognizing his talent first, he may not have ended up being the gifted composer he is today. If you stop and think about it, there may be things in your life that you have consistently received compliments on. What are they? If you can't think of any, don't be discouraged.

Ask several important people in your life whom you trust and who love you *unconditionally* what they think you are naturally good at doing. Sometimes that can also be an important key to discovering

Energy Girls® Question

What do others compliment you on?

Energy for God's Wome

what we are wired to do and what other things we can add back into our lives to create more energy.

A Certificate Is Not a Gift

It is important that at some point other people acknowledge you have the gift you think you have. How many of us have had at least one teacher in our life who was so motivating, such a great communicator, and so energizing that we could hardly wait to get to class? That teacher had *the gift* of teaching—the golden ability to awaken minds, inspire dreams, and encourage young hearts. Her interest and enthusiasm were boundless.

Unfortunately, we may have also sat through some classes not learning much, perhaps even blaming ourselves, because a teacher with all the right credentials did not have a gift—and should have been doing something else altogether. Not much fun for us, but think of the teacher. She must have been exhausted at the end of each day from trying to spin gold from straw. The fact that you can get a certificate or even a degree doesn't *necessarily* mean you have a gift in that field. So when you're exploring your talents and abilities, keep in mind that other people will see your God-given gifts too.

It's important to face reality if you are going to discover your gifts and have a life filled with energy. You may think you are good at something, really gifted at something, but perhaps you're not. So ask your friends to tell you the truth. Remember question number three? *What do other people compliment you on?* Well, if you're not sure, ask a few of your closest friends. But remember to ask only people you trust and who love you unconditionally, and then try to face reality if no one else confirms you have the gift you think you have. No sense wasting time.

Live Life Fully

Consider what you already know now—that even when you are exhausted and feel like you can't take another step—if someone asks you to do something that utilizes one of your natural gifts, suddenly you *come to life*. You have energy. This sense of excitement, even renewal, is a different kind of energy than the adrenaline rush required to perform extraordinary physical tasks. It's a joy and energy that comes from deep inside your heart.

You may not have given it much thought, but discovering your gifts and then learning how to put them to use is also an essential element in living life to the fullest. It's a joyful, exciting task to find out who you really are in God. I promise, if you commit yourself to it, the benefits will go far beyond what you can imagine, and not the least of these will be *more energy*. You will also discover that you can make decisions more easily, know what tasks you should and shouldn't do, and you will learn how much you have to offer others—gifts that are both important and unique.

How to Give Your Gifts

Much has been written to help people discover the best way to *use* their gifts. For example, some people like to work alone and actually need solitude to restore their energy. For others, being around people is energizing. Some work best at a steady pace; others are far more efficient given a tight deadline. Some of us do our best thinking in the morning; others of us are night owls. The differences go on and on, and learning your own answers to these questions is a wonderful process of discovery. As you answer these questions and learn more about how you were created, you will not only find that you have more energy, but more empathy. Heightened understanding and sensitivity to those around you will result as you gain new insights about how *others* are gifted. You will realize that all the people around you have different abilities, different "wiring," and they, with their differences, might give you just the fresh perspective you need.

All Things Bright and Beautiful

Women are worn out. We often spend all our energy trying to keep up with the fast-paced world around us. Things can feel out of control. Maybe you've felt forced to crowd out everything that makes your life bright and beautiful—the things that keep you naturally energetic. If you are in this kind of predicament, it's imperative that you stop, pray, and assess the situation.

It's all about balance and tipping the scales in the right direction. From experience, I've found that women who learn what their gifts are—and then use them in simple ways throughout the day—have more energy, enthusiasm, and joy for everything else they do.

Women who recognize and use their gifts, talents, and abilities fully can accomplish great things. They are also more accepting and better at working with others because knowing their own gifts helps them understand and appreciate others' gifts more easily.

You, too, can be a woman with a sense of purpose in every situation and not waste your time and energy trying to do things you're *not* gifted to do.

Your Life is More Than Problems

When you are under stress and exhausted, whether at home or in an office, you start to feel that your whole life is nothing but the problems you're facing. You lose perspective. You lose energy. I have spoken with women who are so burdened by one specific problem they're facing that they feel like that problem has taken over their life. But your life is so much more than the stress in your job, a problem in a relationship, or difficulties of any kind. Putting your God-given gifts and talents back into action will give you a broader perspective.

Although we never feel as though we have time to add something to our already busy schedules, sometimes it's just what we need to give us an energy boost and a new, healthier outlook.

I came that they may have life and have it abundantly.
John 10:10 (NASB)

Look Into Your Heart

Think of your gifts as being the broad array of skills, talents, and abilities you possess. How else can you discover what those are? The answer sounds almost too simple—you just look inside your heart.

Energy for God's Women

Dear Best Girlfriend...

Many years ago as a young woman in college, I took a class where we were required to go to a special career development seminar. The seminar was led by Richard Bolles, the well-known author of *What Color Is Your Parachute?*, now the world's most successful and popular book on career development. We were given a simple assignment to help us discover what gifts, interests, and talents we might have, and how we might use them. I was asked to pretend I was writing a letter to a best girlfriend whom I had not seen in five years. The letter was to explain that, during the five years since I had seen her, I had found my *dream* job! Richard Bolles told me to write in detail, outlining every aspect of my new job—nothing was too small. It was not easy to do at first.

I wrote about how much I liked what I did, how my office looked, what kind of people I worked with, where we lunched, what the environment was like—and what it was not like—even what we did hour by hour throughout the day. At the time, as a young woman, I was clueless about what I was supposed to do with my life. However, I was excited by the assignment and found it truly revolutionary to let myself dream *big*. It forced me to look deep into my heart and helped me discover what God might be calling me to do.

You may have heard the question "What would you do if you knew you could not fail?". In this letter the sky was the limit. I wrote it straight from my heart as if it were *impossible for me to fail*. It was not about setting goals—it was about searching my heart and seeing what was there. It was about dreaming big and letting myself imagine things as they might be. Later on, I knew I could create goals and a timeline of what I might need to do to make my dream a reality.

I want to challenge you to write a similar letter. Sit down and write to your pretend best girlfriend as though you were right now living your dream. Maybe your dream is being a mom who home-schools your five kids—and the neighbor kids, too. Maybe your dream job is having a TV talk show, owning a business, becoming a teacher, musician, or artist. There are no right or wrong answers.

I guarantee this will start stirring things up inside you— and if you've given your whole heart completely to Christ, you can also trust that he has put many of his desires in you, for his purposes to be fulfilled in your life.

> **Delight yourself in the LORD; and He will give you the desires of your heart.**
>
> Psalm 37:4 (NASB)

It may not be easy to let yourself dream at first, but I believe you will find within your letter an important *seed of truth* that will help you discover what your God-given gifts are and how you can use them to energize your life and help others.

My life was completely changed by my simple letter. It started to give me a vision for what I was called to do. Today I am doing almost exactly what I wrote in that letter many years ago—except that what I'm doing today is far better because it's all about the Lord and what he wants. I feel he is letting me be a part of his big plan. I

Energy Girls® Tip

How else can you discover your gifts? The answer sounds almost too simple—you just look inside your heart.

have grown beyond the desires I had as a young woman and am doing things now that are more meaningful than I could ever have imagined when I wrote the letter entitled "Dear Best Girlfriend." I have also discovered time and time again that any gifts I have been given are not for me at all, but to use to help and serve others—and that makes all the difference.

Out of Your Pain and Trials

Your experiences in life, both good and bad, also contribute to what you can offer. The hardest thing you have ever faced, the most painful and difficult, can also be a great gift from God. He has promised that he will take what you give him and redeem it.

Experience has taught me that the hardest, most difficult things I've been through have been the things that have given me the very best opportunities to learn about how to use my gifts in the way the Lord intended for me.

When I was a young woman, I was diagnosed with cancer. I didn't know whether I would live or die—but God knew. I'm so grateful he restored my health. Of course, I wouldn't wish what I went through on anyone, but honestly, I wouldn't trade the experience for the world, either. It became a great gift in my life. In that terribly difficult time, I learned about God's faithfulness— and yes, his joy—in a whole new way. I learned that our dreams can be completely broken—even turned to dust—but that Jesus can replace "ashes for beauty" and give us something far better that we could ever imagine. If you ask him, he will use any trials you're in to bring you closer to him—and then he will use your trials as a gift to others.

One of my dearest girlfriends suffered terrible physical abuse as a child. She has taught me a lot about how God can use even the most awful circumstances and turn them around. She is one of the kindest, most compassionate women I know. So often I've seen her reach out to other women who are hurting and give just the right touch of kindness to bring healing to a situation. It's a gift. I know it's because of what she went through. She knows what it is to hurt—and to forgive.

Another girlfriend of mine was simply planting flowers outside of her country church on a Saturday, in the middle of the day, when she was brutally attacked from behind, dragged off, raped and beaten. Somehow she got to the road and hollered for help. She is one of the most courageous women I have ever met. Although small in stature, from the very first moment she was rescued, she fought—with God's help, mercy, and grace—not only to recover and forgive, but to use her terrible attack as a gift to others. She is now a chaplain for other women who have been through similar, horrific experiences.

> *Energy Girls® Fact!*
>
> Your experiences in life, both good and bad, also contribute to what you can offer. The hardest thing you have ever faced, the most painful and difficult, can also be a great gift from God.

What have you been through? Death of a loved one, divorce, failed relationships, children that have gone astray, illness, abuse, financial problems? It doesn't matter what it is, Jesus is our redeemer. Can you see God's hand at work to redeem your situation? If not, he wants to show you that he can do that in your life—no matter what the problem. Your ordeal and trial can be a gift because it can bring you closer to God and mature you, so that in your brokenness and weakness, God can use you more powerfully. He will shine through you. If your heart is broken at this moment, simply ask God to use your brokenness to show you his strength. God loves to use our weaknesses.

The LORD is close to the brokenhearted and saves those who are crushed in spirit.

Psalm 34:18 (NIV)

He gives power to those who are tired and worn out; he offers strength to the weak.

Isaiah 40:29 (NLT)

Perhaps you have been through something so awful you think it's holding you back, keeping you from using your gifts. I believe just the opposite. It might be the very thing that allows you to use your gifts and talents in the most powerful way possible.

It's Never Too Late

Some women never give up. Evelyn Gregory, from North Carolina, wanted to become a flight attendant shortly after World War II. Her father, with the very best intentions, discouraged her interest in flying as a career choice. So instead she got married, had three children and over the years, a successful career at the local bank. She eventually became branch manager but she never forgot what was in her heart—what she really felt called to do.

After her husband passed away and she retired, Evelyn went to live in Myrtle Beach. She divided her time between collecting seashells, visiting with her grandkids, and teaching Sunday school class at nursing homes. And then, decades after God first instilled in her that desire, she decided to apply to become a flight attendant. She was looking for something to do that was more *energizing.*

US Airways turned her down twice, but that didn't stop her. She didn't give up. Evelyn applied again, became a ticket agent, and then applied to become a flight attendant with Mesa Air Group. She was finally accepted.

After attending flight attendant school—where her roommate was only 18—her big day finally arrived. There she was at Charlotte Douglas International Airport, announcing to her passengers on the plane, "You may not believe this but, at age 72, this is my first flight!" When asked later about how she felt about her new adventure, she said, "God has placed me where I need to be. We have a mission in life. If we can do something that is useful to others, I say go for it!"

Fill Your Life with Joy and Energy

Discovering your personal gifts and using them regularly in your work, at home, and in all your relationships will fill your life with renewed joy, purpose, and energy. Even the mundane can suddenly take on new meaning when you recognize you have something special to offer that makes a difference in the lives of others. If you already know what your special gifts and talents are, find a way to use them. If you don't, start taking a journey of discovery that can energize your life.

Your Amazing Gifts – Questions for You to Answer

As you answer the following questions, I hope you will gain new insight. Insight can be the key to growth, change, and developing a vision for what God wants you to do with the gifts he has given you.

Have you ever taken a spiritual gifts test or has someone taught you how to discover your spiritual gifts?

If you answered yes, what is one spiritual gift you are confident God has given you?

If you answered no, what one action step can you take to learn more about your spiritual gifts (i.e., study the scriptures, talk to someone at church, take a spiritual gifts test, etc.)?

Questions...

What do you love to do so much you lose track of time? What excites you and energizes you? Any hobbies, educational pursuits, volunteer activities? Your answer could include anything from cooking to painting, working with animals or encouraging a friend. How can you include those energizing activities in your life?

Have you ever received compliments on a particular activity? Has someone ever said to you, "You're good at that!" What was it? What do you think your strongest abilities and gifts are?

Does that activity also seem to come naturally to you? Is it easy and effortless?

Questions...

If you're busy as a mom, wife, homemaker, teacher, or if you're on any job—how can you use some of your gifts in a small, simple way now, in ways that might give you more energy and enthusiasm for all the other things you do? How can you add a few "bright and beautiful" things back into your life?

What painful experiences have you experienced, and what weaknesses do you have that God might use so you can help others?

If you were assured of success, and you could not fail, what is the one thing you would like to make sure you do before your life is over?

Step 2: Relationship SOS

Love is patient and kind. Love is not jealous or boastful or proud or rude. It does not demand its own way. It is not irritable, and it keeps no record of being wronged. It does not rejoice about injustice but rejoices whenever the truth wins out. Love never gives up, never loses faith, is always hopeful, and endures through every circumstance.

1 Corinthians 13: 4-7 (NLT)

"We should have been there by now," I told my new husband. I was exasperated. A trip that was supposed to take an hour and half was taking more than two hours, with no end in sight. The reason? My husband was on one of his "favorite" back roads. We had been married only a few months and were on our way to see my husband's big family, including his six sisters, all of whom lived in Denver, Colorado.

Our first home was a log cabin and there were plenty of back roads where we lived, high in the Rocky Mountains. I knew it was a real log cabin because I could clearly see the national forest between each log and I had to keep the wood-burning stove lit to stay warm. My husband—one of the original outdoor guys—loved taking back roads, hiking through the forest and doing anything that kept him close to nature. I, on the other hand, was the original mall girl from the suburbs, and my idea of roughing it was taking a walk in a park during the day—and staying at a very nice hotel at night.

It's Always Something

After a few more miles we got into a heated argument. In relationships and especially marriage, it seems it's always the little things that drive you crazy. Clothes not picked up. Toothpaste caps left off. I think it's easier to rise to the occasion for big disasters and, like everyone, we've had our share of those.

Why, I thought, *can't he just take the simplest route?* I didn't know it at the time, but a quick analysis of our situation would have proved the obvious. I was the organized, structured one who liked things direct, to the point. My husband had the exact opposite approach to life. He was laid back, flexible, fun-loving and creative. Brian enjoyed the spontaneity of going a different way to Denver—and seeing the back roads. All the reasons I fell in love with him.

After a few more arguments, we got some help. Since we were newlyweds, we wanted to make sure we learned how to communicate. A friend suggested that we take a personality inventory to help us understand how we were "wired." The results were eye-opening. It showed that, yes, I was wired to feel secure and happy if things were structured, organized, and always the same. My husband, Brian, was happiest when things were spontaneous, creative, and always changing—in other words, when he took the back roads. But the amazing thing we learned should have also been obvious—it said it right there in our assessment—he needed someone just like me to provide order and structure, and I needed someone just like him to keep me flexible and spontaneous. We were the perfect match.

So often, the very things that make a relationship challenging or difficult are also what make it blessed. The bitter with the sweet. Through the good times and the bad, commitment is everything in a marriage relationship. But sometimes the bad times can be very challenging. Ruth Graham, famed wife of the world's great evangelist, Billy Graham, has a wonderful sense of humor. When asked if she ever considered divorcing her husband, she said with a charming smile, "Murder him, yes; divorce him, no!"

And we all know that opposites attract. Brian and I always say there are three things that have helped us over our two decades of marriage. One is forgiving and forgetting seventy times seven—which means daily and regularly. Two, praying to God and asking for help—also daily and regularly. Three, keeping our sense of humor, no matter what. My husband has taught me a great deal about humor. Laughter really is the best medicine, and too often in our relationships we take ourselves far too seriously.

Energy Girls® Fact!

So often, the very things that make a relationship challenging or difficult are also what make it blessed. The bitter with the sweet.

Help! Relationship Energy Drain

There are serious problems in relationships, though, especially in marriage. Some experts say divorce rates are 50 percent, others believe the number is closer to 43 percent, but everyone agrees on one thing: The number of divorces has risen dramatically since 1970, by over 275 percent—a staggering increase. There will be more than a million divorces in the United States this year. That means broken homes, heartbroken family members and complicated relationships with extended and "mixed" families. This, despite the fact that studies and surveys show that Americans actually rank a "happy" marriage higher in importance than anything else—including health, money and job satisfaction.

Women long for unconditional love and intimacy, and we often expect our husbands to meet every one of our needs. No one person can do that, it's not possible. Whether you're single or married, put God first in your life. He's the only one that can truly meet all your deepest needs. Marriage for a lifetime takes work, commitment and prayer. Yet our culture and media still present the idea that all you have to do is find your soul mate, marry them, and then you will live happily ever after. Dr. Neil Clark Warren says, "I believe soul mates are made, not born. You start with the ingredients for a highly compatible, successful relationship, and then you work to develop closeness and intimacy." Couples need to talk more when conflicts arise, and work things out in love. Even more importantly, they need to listen more.

> *Energy Girls' Tip*
> Whether you're single or married, put God first in your life. He's the only one that can truly meet all your deepest needs.

All the women I know are more than happy to talk—and work on relationships. Women tend to make relationships a high priority and often assume the responsibility for everybody's getting along—all of the time. That takes a great deal of energy and also causes an inordinate amount of personal stress and pain in women's lives.

Many people believe that the "no-fault divorce" laws have been a disaster for women, marriage relationships, and the family. Dr. James C. Dobson, founder and chairman of Focus on the Family states, "A person can abandon his or her family more

Energy for God's Women

easily than he can abrogate any other agreement that bears his or her signature. It matters not that he made a solemn promise before God, friends, relatives, a member of the clergy, or a licensed representative of the state. If he changes his mind, he doesn't even have to explain why. Of greatest concern is the welfare of the husband or wife who is unwillingly confronted with divorce, custody battles and rejection. That responsible individual has absolutely no power in the dissolution of the family. But the other spouse, even the person who chases after a younger playmate or a "grand new freedom," is the one in charge."

Whenever I have asked a large group of women if anyone has ever had a relationship that drained them of energy, every hand shoots up and the chorus of "Amens" starts. Women care, and *they care deeply*. And that's why we're so vulnerable when our relationships aren't working.

Violence against women has also increased dramatically, primarily among couples co-habiting. Virginia Wing, an expert who writes on domestic violence, stated, "The act of marriage provides the necessary stability and pledge of endurance required to maintain a healthy intimate relationship...the marriage license is one that demands and affords mutual respect and security." In their book, *No Place for Abuse,* Catherine Clark Kroeger and Nancy Nason-Clark state, "Abuse occurs within every faith community. And it knows no socio-economic boundaries. Rich women, poor women, illiterate women, religious women, beautiful women—all women are potential targets of violence." Clearly, the hurt, pain, and damage this horrific crime causes are immeasurable.

Energy Girls® Fact!

Women tend to make relationships a high priority and often assume the responsibility for everybody's getting along—all of the time.

I enjoy speaking to all kinds of women, and not all of them share my faith in God. Yet, almost without exception, women everywhere will agree there is an alarming increase in immorality today, and it feels like we are living in a world gone mad. Women are overwhelmingly tired and burned out. The breakdown of our families is certainly playing a major role. For women, who are naturally relationship-oriented, this does not bode well, but there is an answer. Dr. Robert Coleman, a renowned Professor of Discipleship and Evangelism, says, "It does look discouraging if you just look at the immorality . . . in our land ... But in the midst of this there's also a great yearning that you find in people, really wanting something that's real, something that's coming alive." You were created for one relationship above all others and you need to restore that relationship first.

There is an Answer

The *one* relationship that will give you hope, help, and be your never-ending energy source in life is your relationship to Jesus. He is the one who made you and he made you to be in fellowship with him—*forever*. He has a plan for you.

> *"For I know the plans I have for you," declares the LORD, "plans to prosper you and not to harm you, plans to give you hope and a future."*
>
> Jeremiah 29:31 (NIV)

If you have a broken heart, if you feel you've been wounded beyond repair, if your dreams for a healthy, whole relationship have been shattered, I have good news for you—God draws near to the brokenhearted.

> *The LORD is close to the brokenhearted and saves those who are crushed in spirit.*
>
> Psalm 34:18 (NIV)

If what you have been through drives you to God, if your broken heart can make you more like Jesus, and if you will allow it to teach you that your relationship to him must be the number one relationship in your life, then no matter what you go through, it will work for your good. I can promise this because—*that's the promise of God.*

> *So, what do you think? With God on our side like this, how can we lose? If God didn't hesitate to put everything on the line for us, embracing our condition and exposing himself to the worst by sending his own Son, is there anything else he wouldn't gladly and freely do for us? And who would dare tangle with God by messing with one of God's chosen? Who would dare even to point a finger? The One who died for us—who was raised to life for us!—is in the presence of God at this very moment sticking up for us. Do you think anyone is going to be able to drive a wedge between us and Christ's love for us? There is no way!*
>
> Romans 8:31-38 (MSG)

> *And we know that God causes everything to work together for the good of those who love God and are called according to his purpose for them.*
>
> Romans 8:28 (NLT)

You may not see it now, but wait. Strong women of God are not made overnight, and the Lord can work changes in your life that will eventually bear great fruit—no matter what you've been through. You can know God's joy in a new way.

> *Weeping may last for the night, but a shout of joy comes in the morning.*
>
> Psalm 30:5 (NASB)

Nothing can separate you from his love—not broken relationships, betrayal by friends, or even your own broken heart.

> *I will never fail you. I will never abandon you.*
>
> Hebrews 13:5 (NLT)

God makes it easy for you to experience all of this; all you have to do is turn your life over to him. Wherever you are and whatever you're doing at this moment, you can just stop and ask him, aloud or silently—he knows, and he will hear you. *Ask Jesus to be the number one relationship in your life and give him your heart.*

> **Look! I stand at the door and knock. If you hear my voice and open the door, I will come in, and we will share a meal together as friends.**
>
> Revelation 3:20 (NLT)

Reality Therapy

When my own spiritual journey began many years ago, I didn't know much about what the Word of God said about relationships. I also had to learn a lot of life lessons the hard way. The very best lesson and the one that has helped me the most, time and time again, is the simple truth that we can't control anyone else's response but our own. That fact is great reality therapy.

You may have relationships that are filled with stress and misunderstanding. Some people are just not easy to get along with. Then again, they may think you're not easy to get along with either! Most women rank conflict in relationships a number one source of stress in their lives every day. The health of women is also effected by stress in relationships, far more than it is for men. A study done at the University of London showed relationship breakups are stressful for both men and women—but women have a much more difficult time getting over the heartbreak, and it's much more detrimental to their mental health. Women need healthy, supportive relationships to thrive. We have all kinds of relationships—as wives, mothers, grandmothers, sisters, aunts, co-workers and friends. It never hurts to go over the relationship basics.

Energy Relationships - Top Ten Tips

1. Experience the Freedom of Forgiveness
2. Be Ready for Conflict
3. Let Go of Your Baggage
4. Get a Mountain-Top View
5. Give Honest-to-Goodness Thanks
6. Make Sure You're Listening
7. Use Communication Basics
8. Hang Out with Truth-Tellers
9. Get Wise Energy Mentors
10. Girlfriend, Keep Laughing!

1. Experience the Freedom of Forgiveness

There is freedom in forgiveness. One thing I've learned over the years is that whenever women hang onto unforgiveness or bitterness, it's extremely draining. It can chip away at the very heart of who you are, without your realizing it. At various times in our lives we might be hurt, misunderstood, or possibly ill-treated. As a woman you might also experience tragedies, crises, or a broken heart. It may be due to your own sin, someone else's, or just the fact that we live in a fallen world. One day it will end—but until then God has told us how we must respond: We need to forgive those who have "done us wrong."

Is there someone you need to forgive? There is a wonderful freedom in forgiveness, and you can experience that freedom *today*. If two women experience the very same tragedy, they might respond differently. One might cast blame, look for revenge, and become very bitter. Another woman might grow spiritually, draw closer to God, and develop greater empathy for others. What is the difference between the two? We know that "The same sun that melts the wax hardens the clay." It all begins with a choice. You must choose to forgive.

You can decide today to let go of any bitterness, hurt, anger or resentment you feel, and turn it over to God. When you study God's Word, it's very clear—Christ actually *commands* us to forgive. It's *not* optional. He said he would forgive us, as we forgive others.

I know many women who also need to forgive themselves—for mistakes made, stupid decisions, wrong choices, hurts they've caused others. Jesus said to the woman caught in sin, "Neither do I condemn you, go and sin no more" John 8:11. Do you need to forgive yourself? God wants to lift that heavy burden from your heart.

The emotional feelings you have may not change right away—but decide you will forgive, no matter what someone has done. Your emotional feelings can catch up later. Forgiving will set you free and release God's healing in your life. Don't let unforgiveness or bitterness drain you of energy.

2. Be Ready for Conflict

There will always be conflict. Don't be surprised when it happens. The question is—are you ready to resolve conflict in a godly, positive way? Conflict is a symptom that communication has broken down. Conflict can also be the catalyst for change, spiritual growth, and an opportunity to develop more honest, real relationships.

Energy Girls® Tip

Forgiving will set you free and release God's healing in your life. Don't let unforgiveness or bitterness drain you of energy.

Often when conflicts happen, people take things personally. Remember, it will help everyone if you focus on the problem and the *solution*—not on any one person.

Often conflicts are complex and will require patience, prayer and wisdom. And don't forget your sense of humor. No one likes conflict. It increases stress and can make people uncomfortable and insecure. But with God's help and your dedication to finding a solution, conflicts can make you a stronger woman of God.

You can be ready for conflict if you:

- Are not surprised when it occurs.
- Remain calm and pray.
- Are willing to listen to the "other side."
- Remain open to compromise.
- Focus on the problem and *solution*—not the person.

3. Let Go of Your Baggage

Have you ever noticed that something that doesn't bother you at all might set someone else into a stress-filled tailspin? You're left wondering, *what are they so upset about?* It may be they have baggage they're still carrying around from past experiences. We all have it. For example, when I was growing up, our family talked easily and naturally about finances. On the other hand, my husband remembers discussions about money that were filled with tension. Guess what happened when we had our first financial discussions? You could cut the tension with a knife, and I didn't know why. Once I learned about my husband's past experiences, I could easily understand it wasn't personal and it wasn't even about us—it was simply baggage.

We all waste far too much energy in relationships trying to prove we're right, and not enough on understanding other people. Most of the time, people are not trying to be difficult; they're just looking at things *differently*. We need to spend more energy on understanding the other person's perspective, experience, and feelings—and far less on proving that we're right.

Is there someone you're having a problem with right now? What past experiences might they have had that make them feel like they do? Knowing the answer to that simple question can be a helpful tool for life-giving, energizing relationships. We've been given new life in Christ. If you're carrying past baggage that's too heavy, with God's help you can let it go.

4. Get a Mountain-Top View

When relationship problems make you feel like you're stuck in a rut, it helps to get a fresh perspective. To work my way through graduate school, I had a very stressful job. I was responsible for hundreds of patients and staff in a long-term health care facility. I was concerned about each and every person, and always found it difficult to leave at the end of my night shift unless each patient received the highest standard of care.

Since we were always short of staff, this level of care was almost impossible. Many times, I left filled with stress and discouragement. We lived right near the mountains, and on my days off, I would drive as far as I could high up in the mountains. By the time I reached the top of the snow-capped Rockies, I saw things differently. By the end of the day I was refreshed and released from my burden, although the situation I found myself in was no different. I felt renewed, energized, and ready to go back down the mountain and get back to work.

What changed? *My perspective.* What relationship situation are you in now that needs a new, fresh perspective—a mountain-top experience? How can you get it? If you don't live near the mountains, maybe you can have your own mountain-top experience by talking to a trusted friend, going on a mini day retreat to seek God, setting up an appointment with a wise, spiritually mature person, or getting professional counseling. When you feel trapped in a draining relationship, it's crucial you step back to see the relationship from a new perspective. That can make all the difference. Your situation may not change—but you will.

5. Give Honest-to-Goodness Thanks

Having a grateful heart will give you energy. It will also add joy to your life. Having a grateful heart can even help restore relationships. No matter what you've been through, there's always something you can be grateful for. There will always be women who have more than you do, and some who have much less. There will always be women who seem to be brighter, prettier, have more perfect kids or nicer homes, or whatever it is you think you want—and those who appear to have almost nothing. Things are never quite what they seem, and I can assure you that no one's life is perfect because there are no perfect people.

I've met very successful women who seem to have it all and are completely miserable—and I've met those who, by this world's standards, appear to have almost nothing, and yet they are completely joyful. What's the difference? A grateful heart.

> **Be thankful in all circumstances, for this is God's will for you who belong to Christ Jesus.**
>
> 1 Thessalonians 5:18 (MSG)

Whenever you're grateful, you become thankful. When you're thankful, you start praising. And when you start praising, you're lifted up and you experience God's joy—and the joy of the Lord is your strength.

It's so easy to focus on all the negatives in relationships. They will always be there if you look for them. And once you go down that road, it seems to feed on itself. Focus instead on anything positive you can. We are all a mixture of good and bad, and there's always good we can find in everyone. Right now, if you're in a challenging relationship, start to cultivate some honest-to-goodness gratefulness and see what happens. If you honestly don't have any, simply ask the Lord to change your heart and give you a grateful one.

> **I will praise you, Lord, with all my heart; I will tell of all the marvelous things you have done.**
>
> Psalm 9:1 (NLT)

6. Make Sure You're Listening

Listening can solve problems and conflicts before they escalate. Some hair stylists are really great listeners and they often dispense comfort, sympathy, and advice. Why is it women open up their heartaches and heartbreaks to their hair stylists? I think "girl talk" happens naturally in certain settings. My friend and hair stylist, Mona, was so good at listening to her clients—and offering practical help and guidance—she became a marriage counselor.

Mona has been a pastor's wife for many years. Her husband pastors a large church, and together they started successfully counseling couples years ago. She gave me three golden insights the Lord has shown her through many hours of helping others. First, she thinks the most important challenge in a relationship is listening. She says we don't listen to what is being said because we get caught up in our own agenda. Second, not listening can create serious problems when we're trying to communicate love, caring, and concern; and third, when we care more about our agenda than the other person's, we can't listen and learn *what not to do*. And knowing what not to do may be just as important.

The wrong way to communicate in the middle of a conflict is through belittling, criticizing, stonewalling, or escalating a problem. Instead, create a safe environment to share in—a place where trust and listening and openness are actively pursued. Next time you face a conflict, before you're completely drained of energy, ask yourself: What can I do to be an active listener? What can I do to create a safe environment for someone else? Take small steps to improve your listening skills, and it will create big energy rewards—in all of your relationships.

7. Use Communication Basics

We have dozens of casual relationships, and sometimes we forget the communication basics. Constantly having to repeat information because you're not heard or understood the first time can drain you of energy. Whether you're in the workplace, your community, or in your neighborhood, you have to communicate in a variety of ways all day long.

I grew up in a family of communicators. My Dad was in television and radio and was also a successful columnist for a major newspaper. He was a great communicator. I hope I learned a few things growing up in that environment. When I began my own career, I spent time every week speaking to people from every imaginable socio-economic background and giving health information to the general public on both radio and television.

I was surprised so many people seemed to ignore the communication basics. Studies actually show "workplace civility" has gone downhill in the last decade. And everyone knows it's draining and stressful when you're not treated kindly. One study showed human resource managers ranked communication problems as the number one cause of stress in the workplace. How do you exchange information with people hour by hour and keep your daily interactions full of energy? Since all healthy relationships are based on honest and effective communication, even casual relationships can benefit from effective, thoughtful communications.

Try these easy, simple, energizing communication tips, but remember that you can't control others people's communication habits—only your own.

✓ Make sure your non-verbal cues match your words. Studies show that 80 percent of communication is actually non-verbal.

✓ Greet people warmly. Smile when you see them, and use their name. Everyone loves the sound of their own name.

✓ When you're busy, don't act like it. Instead, act and speak *calmly*. Stay focused on the person you are speaking to and give them your undivided attention—even if your heart's racing, the clock is ticking and you have a deadline looming.

✓ Anticipate questions in conversations—and answer them before they are asked.

✓ Restate what someone tells you, so they know they have been heard.

✓ When you need to have an important conversation, dress the part. Dress in a way that enhances your credibility and inspires confidence in others.

8. Hang Out with Truth-Tellers

When you have a relationship challenge, nothing is more helpful than a friend who will speak the "truth in love." The last thing you need when you're struggling in a relationship is someone who tells you, "You're right, it's hopeless!" You need truth-teller girlfriends who can see beyond your current predicament—still believe God's Word—and hold you to a higher standard. Do you have girlfriends like that in your life? You're blessed if you do. If you don't, start cultivating friendships that will provide you with the truth when you need it most. Use discretion in deciding whom you will get advice from, because the wrong advice is always an energy enemy that can leave you feeling hopeless and helpless.

Advice from a truth-teller spoken in love can help you grow—give you energy—and bring healing to a challenging relationship situation by getting you back on the high road.

9. Get Wise Energy Mentors

To be energized in relationships, you need wise energy mentors. The culture around us does not promote healthy relationships. If you turn on the TV, read magazines or look to Hollywood for advice, you may be sorry. You need to build a positive support network that will inspire you to be God's woman.

Don't limit yourself. As women, we have a lot to offer each other—think intergenerationally. I've been working with one of my dearest friends and professional colleagues, Tina, for more than 15 years. There is quite an age difference between us but we think it works to our advantage. Time and time again, we have seen God use our fellowship to keep us both on track and be a blessing to others. I'm the older, she's the younger, but we each have a unique perspective because of that difference. We are passionate about helping other women do their best. We want to inspire God's women and help them live a healthier lifestyle.

Muriel, my next-door neighbor for years, was an inspiration and energy mentor to me. She always offered me wise counsel, great insight, and the wealth of many years of experience. She was my dearest friend. When I was talking to her one day about the Energy Girls® Network we were creating, she—at the age of almost 90—didn't miss a beat and said with a twinkle, "I'm an Energy Girl!" She recently passed away, and one of the greatest blessings of my life was being able to pray with her in the last hours of her life, before she went home to be with the Lord. I miss her terribly.

If you're hanging out with women who do nothing but gossip, backbite and tear others down, you'll be drained of energy in no time. The best way to deal with it? *Don't do it!* You can be the one to make a difference at work, at home, or wherever you go. Create energizing, godly relationships by being the most loving, kind, encouraging woman you can be, and watch what a difference it makes and how energized you become in the process. Live by the highest standards based on God's Word. Then get with other women who want the very same thing and tell them to hold you to your commitment.

You can't make it alone. Pray and ask God to help you develop Energy Mentors that will encourage you or, better yet, join the Energy Girls®.

10. Girlfriend, Keep Laughing!

It's great to laugh. Most of my life, I've been told I'm a serious person—but not anymore. The Lord gave me one of the funniest guys on earth for a husband. Now people tell me I'm pretty funny. If so, I owe it all to my husband, Brian. He has never let me take myself too seriously—and it's a good thing because laughter is good medicine and, like all women, I need more of it.

> **A joyful heart is good medicine.**
>
> Proverbs 17:22 (NASB)

Published studies have shown that laughing lowers blood pressure, reduces stress, boosts our immune system, decreases pain and, of course, gives women a general sense of well-being. Even in tragic situations I have seen many women use a touch of humor to lighten the load and lift everyone's spirits. It also helps to get our minds off an immediate crisis and gives us a much-needed break.

Laughter is a gift, an energizing relationship tool, and one that might make you more resilient when relationship challenges come. Or as Eleanor Roosevelt said, "A woman is like a tea bag. You never know her strength until you drop her in hot water!" So, girlfriend, next time you feel like you're being dropped in hot water—*keep laughing!*

Relationships Can Fill Us with Endless Energy

Energy Girls® Tip

Ultimately—and this is good news—you can control only one thing in any relationship: Your own response. That simple truth can make all the difference.

When relationships are full of joy and are supportive and affirming, they have the ability to fill us with an energy that seems endless. On the other hand, when relationships are filled with mistrust, hurt, anger or bitterness, nothing can be more draining. Ultimately— and this is good news—you can control only one thing in any relationship: Your own response. That simple truth can make all the difference. But the most important thing is to build every relationship in your life on the foundation of the one and only relationship you were created for—your relationship to God.

Step 3: Declutter Your Life

Then, turning to his disciples, Jesus said, "That is why I tell you not to worry about everyday life—whether you have enough food to eat or enough clothes to wear. For life is more than food, and your body more than clothing. Look at the ravens. They don't plant or harvest or store food in barns, for God feeds them. And you are far more valuable to him than any birds! Can all your worries add a single moment to your life?"

Luke 12:22-25 (NLT)

Do you want to do something about the clutter in your life but have trouble doing it? Is it robbing you of the energy you need for far more important things? Clutter *is* robbing women of energy, and it's a big, big issue. Women need a place where they can rest. A place where they can find peace. We can't find peace at home when there's "stuff" everywhere—and most women feel guilty as the piles continue to grow. At best, clutter becomes an energy drain; at worst, it's completely immobilizing.

When I first explained to someone that I was going to speak on "How to Declutter Your Life," my friend said,

"Oh, you mean emotional clutter and stuff like that?" I said, "No. I mean the stuff in your closets, drawers, and the piles around your house!"

We are overwhelmed with *things*. Some studies suggest that women can be wasting as much as 40 percent of their daily energy dealing with household clutter. There are a few women for whom this is not an issue—emphasis on *few*. I used to room with one. She was a college roommate I will never forget. The first time I saw her closet I was impressed. Every single shoe was in perfect alignment, and all her clothes were hung on color-coded hangers. Her purses were on special hooks, and her sweaters were folded to perfection. "Wow!" I said, "You are so organized. How do you keep up with that?" She looked at me blankly and said, "Keep up with *what*?" I knew at that moment we were very different.

I actually enjoy organizing things, but then somehow everything seems to rapidly disorganize, and I have to reorganize again and *again*. Have you ever felt that way? My roommate, on the other hand, *always* had things organized. She could have created the motto *There's a place for everything and everything in its place*. Clutter was never an issue for her. I also know at least one woman who's so organized she has all her spices alphabetized in her kitchen cupboard. I'm glad there are a few of you out there. God bless you. *This chapter is not for you!* However, I bet you have a friend or two who could use this information.

Energy Girls® Fact!

Clutter is robbing women of energy, and it's a big, big issue. Women need a place where they can rest. A place where they can find peace.

DO YOU LIVE IN CLUTTER LAND?

What does your clutter level say about you? Do you live in Clutter Land? Are you making choices that increase your daily clutter and drain you of energy? Or do your choices help you create a peaceful, restful home and workspace?

Answer these simple questions and find out. For each question, simply answer Yes or No.

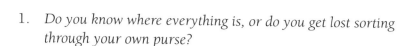

1. *Do you know where everything is, or do you get lost sorting through your own purse?*

2. *Does clutter seem to appear out of nowhere and multiply all by itself?*

3. *Have you been saying for more than a year, "I'll take care of that tomorrow?"*

4. *Does it look like a hurricane hit your drawers and closets?*

5. *Would you mind if your girlfriends opened all your kitchen cupboards?*

6. *Do you dread dealing with your current clutter situation?*

7. *Are you overwhelmed by the piles you see everywhere?*

8. *Are you bleary-eyed from opening junk mail?*

9. *Do you have one space to retreat to that is always clutter-free?*

10. *Do you frequently come across things and say, "I wondered where that was!"*

11. *Do you have less and less uncluttered space and more and more stuff?*

12. *Do you feel like you live in Clutter Land and you need a one-way ticket out?*

Too Much Stuff

I've discovered a simple plan that will help you successfully deal with clutter. My action plan is based on three simple steps. I know this plan can work for you because it works for me, and I'm not "organizationally gifted" like my roommate with the color-coded hangers—and I probably never will be. Before we begin to declutter our lives, however, we first need to look at how we got to the place of having so much stuff and why it has now become a huge issue in our lives. Remember, when the clutter is finally conquered, women can experience renewed energy.

Picture this: You arrive home after a busy day. You try to gather all the mail which is falling out of your hands because of the never-ending "junk" mail that grows in your mailbox. When you sort through it, you toss most of it away. Then, to prepare dinner, you use pre-packaged, processed items because you're short on time, and that also produces more trash to be thrown away. Next, you race to the store and purchase the kids some items for school. When you open the packages, you discover most of the wrapping has nothing to do with the item itself—it's all packaging materials, once again, to be thrown away. We have more trash than ever before. Every day, the average woman (and man) in this country produces about four pounds of trash—that's around 1,460 pounds of trash per person every year.

That's not true everywhere, however. My husband and I planned a special trip to London for our 25th anniversary. It was the trip of a lifetime. We had never been overseas before, and it's funny the little things you notice when you're in a new culture for the very first time. When we arrived in London, we checked into our hotel and decided to go for a walk. We stayed right by Buckingham Palace and St. James Park. We stopped by a "lunch cart" in the park, grabbed a bite to eat and kept on strolling and sight-seeing. When we finished eating, I wanted to throw away the wrapper from my sandwich but couldn't find a trash bin. *How odd*, I thought, *there are no trash containers around.* We kept walking, and still no trash containers anywhere. *There must be a trash can somewhere,* I kept thinking. Eventually, we found one. But we had to walk long and far to find it. This was one of the first things I noticed in the UK—they have less trash and very few trash bins. Here, we have huge trash containers everywhere, every few feet if you need one. More trash always equals more *clutter.*

Disposable Income Equals More Clutter

In the 1940s and 1950s, our buying power changed dramatically in this country. All of a sudden, people had more disposable income, and that was especially true of the middle class. More disposable income meant everyone could buy more disposable goods, and more disposable goods meant *more disposable clutter.*

Today, we also have credit offered and used on a scale unheard of in any other generation. The very first credit card was "Diners Club," and it was created in 1950. In the first year, 20,000 cards were distributed. Today, there are more than 1.5 *billion* credit cards used, and that number continues to grow. The average woman has between five and ten cards in her wallet.

In decades past, if items could not be paid for with cash outright, people just did without; consequently, they had less stuff. Today, it's a rare woman who doesn't have multiple credit cards to make purchases and who hasn't been stressed out at some time in her life with the additional fees, costs, and overbuying that credit card use promotes. We have more than $850 billion in credit card debt, and women make most of the purchases.

Since women today also make more than 80 percent of the buying decisions, marketers and businesses now cater their advertising to appeal to us. They are trying to encourage us to buy more "stuff" by creating credit cards with design and style. Now we have hot pink credit cards, cards with textures that add pizzazz when we pull them out to make purchases—even cards that double as picture frames. Advertisers and marketers have given a name to this strategy—it's called the "Plunk Factor," and it's a credit card designed to make women feel great when they "plunk" the card down on the counter to buy something. When it comes to producing more clutter and more debt, the plunk factor is *not* a good thing.

That Day Will Never Come

Another problem that produces more clutter is that we hang onto things we might use "one day." You know, that magical day in the future when we *really* will have time to repair or fix the one broken item that up to now has been gathering dust. The sheer amount of stuff we buy is ever-increasing, as is how much stuff we throw away—and how much stuff we buy all over again.

Let's say your DVD player is broken. You go to a sale to get a new one. You don't want to throw the old one away because you might repair it—one day. So it goes in the attic or closet, along with the other broken small kitchen appliances that might get fixed but are now gathering dust. But you're too busy to deal with those, so you keep putting things on top of things, and now you want to deal with it

Energy Girls® Fact!

The sheer amount of stuff we buy is ever-increasing, as is how much stuff we throw away—and how much stuff we buy all over again.

even less because it's a big mess. Today, bigger is better, bigger cars, bigger homes, bigger TVs—and *more* is even better than bigger— but all of that contributes to an ever-growing amount of clutter.

In a marriage, it seems that one partner always ends up being the *let's-hang-onto-this* person while the other becomes the *let's-toss-it* person. Sometimes it can be a tug of war. My husband, Brian, usually likes to hang onto things more than I do. One day when I arrived home, Brian was excited and said, "I got something today—it was a great deal and they just need a little fixing, come see." He led me into the garage and I stared in disbelief. There were more than a dozen pieces of wood furniture in all shapes of disrepair. The furniture was stacked as high up as it could go. There was no way we could even put the car in the garage.

I could understand this purchase because my husband loves wood. He loves working with wood, analyzing wood, smelling wood, and being around wood. It's a guy thing. As a young man, he was a carpenter. I, of course—ever the practical one—said, "Do you really have time to repair this stuff?" He assured me that he would find the time. His enthusiasm won me over.

Years later when we were moving and the wood furniture— stacked as high as ever—had never been repaired, he finally saw the light and decided it was time to give all of it to someone who had the time to use it and repair it. To be fair to my sweet husband, I've done the same thing myself more times than I can count, and Brian has helped me realize when it was time to get rid of what I was hanging on to. We help each other.

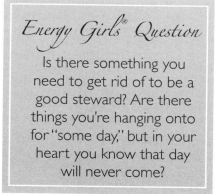

Energy Girls® Question

Is there something you need to get rid of to be a good steward? Are there things you're hanging onto for "some day," but in your heart you know that day will never come?

Is there something you need to get rid of to be a good steward? Something you have an emotional attachment to that you know, deep down, you're probably never going to use again? Are there things you're hanging onto for "some day," but in your heart you know that day will never come?

Who Has the Time?

The overwhelming busyness of women's lives also contributes to the clutter problem. Women are on the go from morning to night, so there's no one home to deal with clutter. Or, they may be at home, but busy all day as a mom or home-business owner. In working with thousands of women over the years, I've found that every woman I know feels responsible at home for all the to-do's, no matter how many jobs she has. The problem is, when a woman is working all day or night, she's rightfully too tired to take care of "things," and her most important responsibility—being the best wife and/or mom she can be—takes priority over everything. And, of course, that's exactly the way it should be. But the problem is that the clutter never gets dealt with.

Energy Girls® Fact!

Women are having a difficult time finding rest and peace because they are on the go every minute, and have very little energy to deal with what they truly care about. They're just trying to keep up with their dizzying array of checklists, things to do, and places to be.

A few decades ago, women were home more. Not as many women were working outside the home, stores were not open 24/7, kids weren't going to a gazillion activities after school and on the weekends. Some things have changed for the better; some have not. More and more women I know are having a difficult time finding rest and peace because they are on the go every minute, and have very little energy to deal with what they truly care about. They're just trying to keep up with their dizzying array of checklists, things to do, and places to be. There's no time or energy left to deal with clutter.

As God's women, we're supposed to be in the world but not *of it*. The culture is going one way; we're to go another. But we're bombarded every day with messages via radio, TV, magazines and the Internet—the message is *buy, buy, buy*. The message is you need more *things*. It's hard not to succumb. It is complicating our lives and it has become a real burden. We need to remind each other that we're supposed to go God's way. Maybe if we lived a simpler life it would help. It's something to think about—something to pray about.

> **And why worry about your clothing? Look at the lilies of the field and how they grow. They don't work or make their clothing, yet Solomon in all his glory was not dressed as beautifully as they are. And if God cares so wonderfully for wildflowers that are here today and thrown into the fire tomorrow, he will certainly care for you.**
>
> Matthew 6:28-30 (NLT)

God Wants to Help

Once when I was nine years old and sleeping over at my best girlfriend's house, her Mom came to tuck us in. She was a lovely sweet woman, and I can still remember clearly what she said as she walked out and closed the bedroom door. "Say your prayers, but don't bother God with your requests. He's too busy!" As I snuggled under the covers, I was very sad. I wasn't sure there was a God but if there was, I was sorry to hear how busy he was because I wanted to talk to him about a lot of things.

As a little girl, I believed God was too busy to be concerned about the details of our lives, but *now* I know that God wants to help us with all our burdens. He wants to have a relationship with us. That means you can talk to him all day long about all the concerns on your heart.

> *O Lord, you have examined my heart and know everything*
> *about me. You know when I sit down or stand up. You*
> *know my thoughts even when I'm far away.*
>
> Psalm 139:1-2 (NLT)

> ## Energy Girls® Tip
>
> God is never too busy for you. He wants to be involved with all of your decisions and he wants to help you in every area of your life. He wants you to pray to him about everything.

God is never too busy for you. He wants to be involved with all of your decisions and he wants to help you in every area of your life. He wants you to pray to him about *everything*. As silly as it may sound, "everything" even includes your clutter.

Ask for his help in dealing with it. I have seen many women so distraught about this issue that it's actually keeping them from doing what God has called them to do. Keeping them from the important things they *should* be doing. That's why I think it's an issue that deserves our time and attention. Besides, the bottom line is that dealing with all this stuff and all this clutter is making the women of America very tired.

Dumpster Saturday

"Ruth, you really need to deal with these piles!" Both my husband and friends had lovingly said the same thing. I knew it was true and I was embarrassed by the situation. I'm not sure how it got to this state, but clutter was everywhere. What made it worse was that I had always prided myself on my organizational abilities, even though now and then my "working" piles of stuff could get out of hand.

I know when it started. I had been in the hospital and hadn't fully recovered my strength or energy. First one pile, then another and another accumulated and, before I knew it, the piles turned into downright obstacles. I ignored the situation. Then it got worse and worse—which made me want to deal with it less and less. I was in *Clutter Land* and couldn't get out.

Then I thought, "OK, I'm going to deal with this, Lord, and if I can learn anything that might help other women, I will be very happy." Dumpster Saturday was born.

I decided to rent a dumpster for the weekend and begin by throwing out all the junk—just tossing it out. Then I would give away items that might help others and, finally, I would store the rest of the clutter away. My hope was that renting the dumpster would jumpstart the entire process. I knew it would cost money to rent it, but I reasoned that the clutter was costing me money too—with lost productivity, lost peace of mind, and constant stress. I decided it would be well worth it.

I also decided to make it fun. I created a "Dumpster Saturday" flyer and posted copies of it around the house. We also made sure we were organized and prepared in advance for every contingency. We got extra packing and cleaning supplies, garbage bags, tape, labels, scissors, and boxes. We made lunch ahead of time and called the Salvation Army and Habitat for Humanity to see what they would take—and what they wouldn't. We set a pick-up time with both of those groups so we knew exactly when they would be coming to get the stuff we were sure we would be giving away.

I even let our neighbors know what we were doing, so they wouldn't be surprised when the dumpster arrived. Actually, this turned out to be the best way we'd ever found to make new friends in our neighborhood. Neighbors we hadn't seen in years got involved, as well as ones we'd never even met. They all stopped by and asked if they could also put a few things in the dumpster. We couldn't believe everyone's response. Several said, "I've thought about doing this, but I'm glad *you* actually did it!" Others laughed with us, and together we all realized we have too much stuff and it just might be a good idea if we considered simplifying our lives and being better stewards.

There was one contingency I couldn't prepare for that did cause some tension, though, and that was deciding what would go in the dumpster—and what wouldn't. We found ourselves going back and forth on some items, kind of like, "should we or shouldn't we?" Without a doubt, "one's man junk is another man's treasure" or, in this case, one woman's. If a family member is not ready to let something go, it might be best not to force the issue.

What actually went in our dumpster? Here's a sampling: Empty paint cans, broken chairs and other furniture, old garden equipment, yard waste, empty computer boxes, broken mattress and box spring, clothes torn way beyond repair, broken hangers, broken sports equipment, torn purses, broken locks, lamps with no bases, broken brooms, pieces of luggage without handles— you get the picture. Just your average run-of-the-mill *junk*.

At the end of the day we not only had a full dumpster, but dozens of boxes, bags, and piles to give away to the Salvation Army and Habitat for Humanity. Best of all, we had order in the house. I felt like a new woman.

The entire event was a huge success, and I would do it again in a minute. Renting a dumpster may not be the best idea for everyone, but I found it to be incredibly motivating. If you ever want to consider "Dumpster Saturday" at your house, here are a few tips I learned:

Dumpster Saturday Tips

- Check around and get bids from several dumpster companies because costs vary—a lot. Use one that offers a flat rate only.
- Make sure you understand what you're allowed to put in the dumpster. Example: Empty paint cans might be OK while full paint cans might not be acceptable.
- Before your actual dumpster day, assess ahead of time what areas you want to declutter, and have a written plan. Allow more time for everything than you think you will need.
- Call the places you want to give items to, see what their policies are for drop-off or pick-up. We like to use the Salvation Army and Habitat for Humanity.

Do What Works for You

Since renting a dumpster is not for everyone, the principle to remember is to do what works for *you*. Maybe that means simply getting another trash can, borrowing a truck to haul a few things away, or buying heavy-duty garbage bags and setting aside a special day to declutter a room. You could also have a garage sale, take your items to a resale or consignment shop, give them to a friend, or sell them on eBay. There are also now full-time "junk removal" companies that specialize in one thing—hauling your clutter away. Do the best you can with what you've got, and be creative. Just remember, however you do it, *less clutter equals more energy.*

Caution: Relationship Alert

Don't force or expect others to immediately share your enthusiasm for decluttering your life. Instead, let them be inspired by your commitment and success. Remember, "Love is patient and kind. Love is not jealous or boastful or proud or rude. It does not demand its own way" (1 Cor. 13:4). Many exasperated women have told me that they've been trying to get rid of junk for years, but their husbands won't let the piles of clutter go and they don't know what to do. First, *pray.* Sometimes God asks us to be patient and wait, and as soon as we give up trying to change another person and love them instead, amazing things can happen. In the meantime, the Lord might just change your heart, too. Please, *don't nag.* I can tell you from experience that nagging never, ever, works. Don't do it.

Energy Girls® Question

Do the best you can with what you've got, and be creative. Just remember, however you do it, less clutter equals more energy. What is the main source of your clutter?

Let's Get Started

So, how can you begin to deal with *your* clutter problem? The first step is to assess *your* current situation. Simply walk around your home and get a feel for just how cluttered your living and work spaces are. If you're fortunate enough not to have a problem with clutter, consider what you might do to simplify and organize your storage spaces to conserve even more energy. Remember, this is a process—you didn't get overwhelmed with clutter overnight,

Energy for God's Woman

and you won't fix the problem overnight either. Start thinking in terms of understanding why the situation is the way it is in the first place and how you really can change it—one pile at a time.

Answer one important question: *What is the main* source *of your clutter?* Is it clothes, toys, magazines, papers, unopened junk mail, closets or drawers that are bulging, or do you run a home-based business that has overtaken your living spaces? Is it items that need repair, or too many items that you just don't need? Whatever your situation, say to yourself, "I can do this. I'm not alone. Clutter, you've had your day!" Remember that there are really two issues here: What caused your clutter problem in the first place, and what you can do to get rid of it now.

Energy Girls® Question

What caused your clutter problem in the first place, and what can you do to get rid of it now?

Action Plan Based on Three Simple Steps

I like things that are simple and to the point. My action plan for decluttering is very simple and it's based on three steps.

Three Simple Steps

1. **Throw it away**
2. **Give it away**
3. **Store it away**

1. Throw It Away

When I first started dealing with my own piles of clutter, I realized I was overwhelmed. It felt immobilizing. I would look at the piles and didn't know where to start. Then I decided I would simply go through the first pile and do *nothing* but straighten up a few things and throw a few things away. It worked. I felt less immobilized and it helped me move forward. I only threw away things I *knew* were "toss away" items. If I was dealing with piles of paper, that might mean junk mail. If I was going through my kitchen drawers, that might mean things way beyond repair.

Now, I do believe in recycling and, being a good steward, I know there's a great deal of guilt in some people about throwing anything away. So if you can recyle and reuse something—go for it, you should do it. But look at it this way: If you're so guilt-ridden about trying to find a use for all your junk that you can't throw out *anything*, and it sits forever gathering dust and causing you stress, what's the point? Besides, no one else may want your junk either—even if you try to give it away. The Salvation Army and other reputable donation agencies have standards. They don't take things beyond reasonable repair and they will tell you that. So, if they won't take something, and it can't be recycled, toss it. It's time to move on.

Caution: Throw It Away Alert

Obviously, many things are one-of-a-kind items, never to be thrown away. For example, I have saved every card my husband has ever given me—for every occasion—over two decades of marriage. I would *never* throw those out. You may have saved all of your children's special mementos. Don't mindlessly throw things away that can never be replaced. Protect those "heart tug" items that are truly a part of your family's history. Most of our clutter is not made up of those things, though, so use common sense.

2. Give It Away

After you throw away all the toss-it items, the next step is "give it away." I'm speaking now about stuff we find in our closets, drawers, cupboards, etc. Obviously, all our office and paper clutter is an entirely different matter.

As you go through things you don't need anymore, set aside anything you want to give to others or put it in a special "Giveaway Box." A good rule of thumb is, if you haven't used something in six months and it's not a seasonal item, do you really need it? Perhaps you could be a good steward by letting someone else use it instead.

When I first started giving away things I wasn't using, there was a tug in my heart over some items, but it got easier and easier, and then it actually became fun. I started giving away some things I was currently using because I felt someone needed them more than I did. There's a freedom in giving things away. As Jesus said, "It is more blessed to give than to receive" (Acts 20:35).

3. Store It Away

Once you've tackled one pile after another and decided what to throw away or give away, it's time to decide what you want to store away. It's a wonderful idea to store things that you don't use daily and weekly. If you haven't used something in three months, store it away and then you will have a clutter-free environment until you're ready to use those items. Women tell me all the time they have more energy when there's less clutter in their living spaces.

Two Store It Away Tips

- Try to store things away so you have empty space on top of key surface areas. That includes kitchen countertops, desktops, dresser tops, etc. You won't believe how much better you will feel if you just look at space that's empty and free of clutter. Do one area and see how you feel. It works.

- It's simpler if you use uniform boxes that are easy to move, such as "banker boxes" with lift-off lids (available in any office supply store). These work well because they can be easily stacked in very small storage spaces. They are also kind on your back when you're lifting, plus you can put a clearly marked label on the outside of each box.

Caution: Store It Away Alert

Because everyone has so much junk today, there are more and more options to store things away at storage centers where you're charged a monthly fee. Also, you can now have a personal storage unit brought to your house and then carted away and stored for you. That may work, but it may also cause you to hang onto stuff you don't need and postpone decisions about decluttering. It will also cost extra money. If you can have less stuff instead of needing a storage unit, it's probably a better idea. Besides, it will take more energy for you to deal with your clutter if it's in a completely different location. Everyone's situation is different, of course, so the most important thing is to do what works best for you.

Hoarding: A More Serious Problem

For a few women, there's an even more serious, deeper problem: "Compulsive hoarding." Such women can't let their clutter go— ever. Their homes are filled with so much clutter that one can barely find space to sit down. This affects their ability to live and work, so much so that they have trouble functioning.

Dr. David Tolin, a specialist in this area, says, "Many people with compulsive hoarding do not recognize how bad the problem really is; often, it is a family member who is most bothered by the clutter." This is considered by many experts to be an obsessive-compulsive disorder that may affect as many as two million Americans. If you suffer from this problem, don't suffer alone because there is help. See a professional, if you need it.

Energy Girls® Declutter Quick Tips

• Keep It Simple

Break overwhelming projects down into smaller projects. Instead of thinking about decluttering your bedroom, think about decluttering just the closet in your bedroom first—nothing else. Breaking the whole thing down into smaller, simpler tasks will make the job easier to deal with.

• Have Simple, Clear, Measurable Goals

Simple, clear goals will keep you from feeling overwhelmed and will give you a feeling of accomplishment. Measurable goals will also keep you focused and help you measure your success. For example, "By Saturday at 5:00 p.m., I will declutter the two kitchen cupboards next to the oven."

• Remember the Closet Rule

The "Energy Girls® Closet Rule" states that each woman's closet has plenty of items, but she generally wears only 20 or 30 of them (her favorite ones, of course) So, why are your closets bulging with so much more? Clothes will come and go. The garments you're hanging onto with the hope that they might, one day, come back in style—won't. And if they did, you probably wouldn't wear them anyway. How about your thin and fat clothes? The ones that you need for all the ups and downs in your weight? The same rule applies. If you're waiting to lose weight, how long have you waited? When that day comes, will the clothes even be in style? When in doubt, throw those clothes out or donate them to someone who can wear them now.

• You Don't Have to Do It All at Once

If one pile is particularly overwhelming, first just straighten it up, throw away anything that's obvious—then take a break. You don't need to do everything at once. When you come back to your pile the second time, start organizing. If it takes several attempts on one pile, that's fine. If you need to break down one, big, overwhelming pile into several small piles, that will also help. Remember: All your clutter didn't appear overnight and you don't need to make it disappear overnight either.

• Get a Girlfriend to Help

Get a girlfriend to help—one you completely trust who is also a natural organizer and let-it-go person. Seeing things from her perspective can help you make decisions more quickly. It's also more fun to share the load with a friend, so you don't feel alone with all your clutter.

• Be Well-Rested and Well-Fed

Make sure you're well-rested before you take on a big declutter project—it won't feel so overwhelming that way. Also make sure you've had something nutritious to eat, for extra energy. Decluttering can be stressful and you need to be at your best to deal with the problem head-on.

- ## Clutter-Free Zone

Women respond to their environment. Create something beautiful in place of the clutter and you will be able to rest and have more energy. Designate one area in your home—even if it's only a corner in a room—to be your personal "clutter-free zone." After it has been set up and decluttered, put something special there to read, such as your favorite magazine, or a book—something to help you revitalize and renew your energy. Replace the space a pile was taking up with fresh flowers.

- ## SOS at Your Desk

It's hard to keep a desk clutter-free. Our desks usually become "paper central" with a mountain of to-do notes. Right now there are probably things on your desk you don't need. Of course you should save (file) truly important tax or business papers. But if you haven't used something in three months, will you ever use it? If not, throw it out. Getting in control of your desk is important for "at-your-desk health." Don't let the paper monster rule.

- ## Your Life on Wheels

A lot of women feel like they live in their cars. Coming and going to work, taking kids here and there, and non-stop shopping to keep hearth and home going. How does your car look right now? It's usually a simple place to declutter because it's not that big. Get your car decluttered and cleaned regularly, and you will feel more energy immediately. Then commit to keeping it that way.

- ## Rest and Have Sweet Dreams

Bedrooms are sacred space to women who are tired. It's the one place I recommend you keep free of clutter at all times. Create a beautiful environment to rest in, so you can have sweet dreams and wake refreshed. When you sleep, your energy is restored. Try to keep piles, laundry, and papers out of your special sleeping spot. How much sleep you need as a woman is unique and individual. The average woman does best with 7-8 hours a night. Since it's so important you get a good night's sleep, use a little ol' fashioned discipline and decide that your bedroom is the one place you will declutter every morning and night. Make it the one place you will keep in perfect order so you can rest.

Remember, It's a Lifestyle

Live a decluttered lifestyle. Simplify things over time and work at developing new, better clutter-control habits each day. Since decluttering is a process, you will need to deal with things *continually*. We will always have to acquire some things—and let others go. It's just a matter of getting more confident that we can manage it all. Some clutter will probably always be with us, so enjoy the journey and keep your sense of humor.

Finally Clutter-Free

For the final step, once you've finished decluttering, add the extras that will make living more enjoyable. Create an environment that is beautiful and restful, one that simply makes you feel good. And don't underestimate the difference this will make in your energy level. Make a statement that says your living space, your work space, and your home are one of a kind. Add fresh flowers, family photos, pictures of inspiring landscapes, or a knick-knack that touches your heart. Create a stress-free, clutter-free, energy-filled environment. You may be a busy, hard-working woman, but you don't have to be drained by clutter to get the job done.

Energy for God's Wom

Step 4: Your Body's Best Friend

Don't you know that your body is the temple of the Holy Spirit, who lives in you and was given to you by God? You do not belong to yourself, for God bought you with a high price. So you must honor God with your body.

1 Corinthians 6:19-20 (NLT)

Your body's best friend is *you*. Your informed, educated, wise decisions can help you have more energy every day. Let me explain.

Like countless other Christians, I believe it's really not about you at all. It's about God and our relationship to him—now and through eternity. That's what matters most. Everything else pales in comparison. As women, we need to have our hearts turned toward our real home. When we get there, we will get new bodies—ones that will last forever. I'm glad, because every day it's obvious to me that the one I'm in now is wearing out!

Do you ever feel you don't measure up? We often feel guilty about our bodies, about how we look and what we eat. We're never quite good enough. It's another reason women are so tired. With God's help, you can apply simple principles that will help you armor yourself against your body's energy enemies. Nothing else can do more for you than making the right daily choices and adopting a healthier lifestyle. The decisions you make about how much you move and what you feed your body make a tremendous difference in your energy level. Since you live inside your body every day, who else should be responsible for it? Until the day you get a new one, why not take care of this body *now*? It's the only one you get. "Don't you realize that your body is the temple of the Holy Spirit, who lives in you and was given to you by God? You do not belong to yourself" I Cor. 6:19 (NLT).

We need to have the right knowledge and information so we can do the best we can with what we've got, and be good nurturers for our families too. That is why I say *you* are your body's best friend. It's your responsibility to make the best choices you can—with all your weaknesses and personal limitations. Accept the fact that in this journey you will make good choices, bad choices and some in-between. The more solid information you have, the more you'll be able to do the right things to give your body energy and, hopefully, reduce your health risks.

> *Energy Girls® Question*
>
> Since you live inside your body every day, who else should be responsible for it? Until the day you get a new one, why not take care of this body *now*?

> *Energy Girls® Tip*
>
> Nothing else can do more for you than making the right daily choices and adopting a healthier lifestyle.

Remember, insight is the key to change. If God wants to give you fresh insight, or even convict you to change something you're doing, great. If, on the other hand, reading this chapter is going to fill you with guilt or condemnation because you already feel you're not measuring up, please stop and pray. God doesn't condemn you.

> *With the arrival of Jesus, the Messiah, that fateful dilemma is resolved. Those who enter into Christ's being-here-for-us no longer have to live under a continuous, low-lying black cloud. A new power is in operation.*
>
> Romans 1:1 (MSG)

Your Amazing Body

Your body is truly amazing. An incredible designer and artist created you. You were made in the image of God. Your life is a gift from God, and your body is a temple of the Holy Spirit. It's hard at work every day, without your even thinking about it.

- Your heart beats about 100,000 times a day and 35 million times a year. Your heart is a pump, and no man-made pump has ever been as reliable.
- Your blood travels 12,000 miles a day—comparable to about three trips across the US, coast to coast.
- Your body breathes in and out more than 23,000 times every day.

God designed your body and it never stops working. It's simple to make choices through the day to help your body along, since it's working hard on your behalf. Any time we talk about women's health, we need to keep it in perspective—God's perspective. If you're anxious and unhappy and you feel your situation is hopeless regarding having more energy or feeling better about your body,

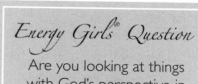

Energy Girls® Question

Are you looking at things with God's perspective in mind, or are you looking at things through the eyes of our current culture?

I have one important question: Are you looking at things with God's perspective in mind, or are you looking at things through the eyes of our current culture? The world's perspective changes constantly and it's impossible to build a solid foundation on it.

Throughout history, women have tried to keep up with the changes. In the 1890s, products were sold to help women "get plump." Fat was in. In the 1960s, super-model Twiggy made anorexia the vogue. Now, in the 21st century, every conceivable inch of a woman's body is under scrutiny, every imperfection noted. Photoshop, digital imaging software, can instantly erase pounds, wrinkles, bad hair days, and less-than-bright white teeth. And what woman can compete with a digital image? It's impossible, in the real world, to live up to the current ideal.

> **Charm is deceptive, and beauty does not last; but a woman who fears the Lord will be greatly praised.**
>
> Proverbs 31:30 (NLT)

Real Women Jiggle

Women's bodies have curves and were made to jiggle. The models we look at constantly have been air-brushed, hair-brushed, and retouched to look like an ideal that simply doesn't exist. Women can't measure up to that and we weren't meant to. Even if you could, through super-human effort, reach your goal of having a perfect body, it would be fleeting. And what does it matter "if you gain the whole world"? Without God in the equation, ultimately there's emptiness at the end of the road.

No matter how many weight loss or fitness programs we try, or how many ways we come up with to keep on the never-ending beauty quest, these bodies of ours will continue to age. They weren't made to last forever but, thank goodness, one day we will get ones that will. After spending years in the field of professional health, fitness and wellness education, I can truthfully say— without a bigger, more selfless view of the whole thing—it's pretty much all "vanity, *vanity*". It's not God's way.

What's a Woman to Do?

So, as God's woman, how can you live with a healthy, hopeful perspective? First, pray and ask God to help you make the right choices, so your body can do what God designed it to do—choices that will give you a sense of well-being and help your body work the way it should, plus restore the energy and joy to your life. There are simple steps you can take to build the right foundation to make those choices easier.

Your body was made to *move*. God designed it that way, but today we're not moving very much. We're sitting in front of our computers, driving everywhere, and engaging in America's favorite leisure activity—watching TV. Everything we do today is easy compared to the work of women long ago. In centuries past, our ancestors had to be physically strong just to survive. "All in a day's work" for a woman meant she had to churn, chop, haul, walk miles to gather wood or food, have a baby, and possibly be back planting crops the next day. Of course, no one wants to go back; childbirth took the lives of many women and infectious diseases were the leading killers of the day. However, the point is that the main health risks women faced were not related to a sedentary lifestyle that resulted in lifestyle-related diseases. By necessity, they got all the physical activity they would ever need in a day.

Today, the number one cause of death for women is heart disease. Now, every year, up to 250,000 American deaths are related to lack of regular physical activity. A recent study showed that in the next decade, America's unhealthy lifestyle will become the number one cause of preventable deaths. James S. Marks MD, MPH and a CDC epidemiologist stated, "We believe diet, inactivity, and obesity—that constellation—will be the leading cause of death if things don't change."

Women who are not physically active are setting themselves up for greater risks for heart disease, high blood pressure, type 2 diabetes, some types of cancers, arthritis, and depression. Depression is a huge issue for women. In fact, women suffer from depression twice as often as men. If women are extremely overweight, they can also suffer from sleep disorders and respiratory problems. Obesity has skyrocketed over the last few decades, and more and more women are now carrying extra weight that's hurting their health. One thing that can't be measured is the toll on women's hearts and minds. But we can do something. It doesn't have to be this way.

If you want to have more energy for all the things God has called you to do, there are important health-related reasons to get motivated, get moving, and start eating right.

Get Moving

Becoming more physically active is God's gift to help you feel better naturally. Women need to get moving. If used safely and effectively, physical exercise will do more for your health and energy level than anything I know. The benefits are tremendous. Studies show that physically active women have fewer hospital stays and physician's visits, and they also use less medication than those who don't remain physically active.

Energy Girls® Fact!

If you want to have more energy for all the things God has called you to do, there are important health-related reasons to get motivated, get moving, and start eating right.

Over the years we've heard tremendous claims by companies who are trying to sell women everything to give them the body of their dreams. If it sounds too good to be true, it is. Trends and buzzwords will always come and go. Build a health-related fitness program on principles that have staying power. Make sure your program can deliver bottom-line results over a lifetime.

By God's grace, I've gained a bit of wisdom over the years, and I've learned time and time again that nothing beats ol' fashioned discipline and consistency to get the job done. There's a way you can add physical activity into your life that's simple and easy, and it will give you more benefits than you can imagine.

BENEFITS OF HEALTH-RELATED FITNESS

You will:

- Have more energy
- Burn more calories
- Decrease the effects of aging
- Have less body fat, more lean tissue
- Feel better about your body
- Strengthen your immune system
- Reduce the chance of depression
- Become stronger
- Improve your bone density
- Sleep more soundly
- Look your best
- Have a heart that works more efficiently
- Reduce your risks for heart disease

1440 Minutes Every Day

You have 1440 minutes each and every day. How many minutes do you think you waste? We could all be better time managers. Considering what's at stake, can you invest a small amount of time in your health? If you took 30 of those wasted minutes, several times a week, and made a commitment to get moving, you would be on the road to having more energy and a new sense of well-being.

"Small, simple steps can often prevent or control chronic health problems such as diabetes, obesity, asthma, cancer, heart disease, and stroke," says former U.S. Surgeon General Dr. Richard H. Carmona. "Prevention includes healthy eating habits and regular physical activity." And that's all it takes, just a few simple steps to make a big difference. Our national guidelines for physical activity state:

- *To improve your health and fitness, get at least 30 minutes of moderate physical activity most days of the week, preferably daily. Greater amounts of physical activity may be necessary for the prevention of weight gain, for weight loss, or for sustaining weight loss.*

Thirty minutes every day is only 2 percent of your time—not much at all. *But it is huge in terms of promoting your health and increasing your energy level.* That small time investment will help you to do what God has called you to the other 98 percent of the time. You will not only reduce your risks for the leading cause of death among women—heart disease—but your bones will be stronger and less brittle and you will have less stress and a brighter outlook on life.

What does "moderate physical activity" mean? If you took a brisk walk and walked about two miles in 30 minutes, that would do it. If you have been living a sedentary lifestyle, you can start by walking just a few minutes a day and work up to one

15-minute mile, then very *gradually* increase your time and distance. You could also break up the 30 minutes into two or three walks during the day of only 10 minutes each. It all counts towards your total goal. Just find a way to be active and stick with it, whether it's walking, attending fitness classes, climbing stairs, pushing a baby stroller, or even gardening.

My older sisters, Carol and Deborah, are walkers. They walk six days a week, rain or shine, sleet or snow. They always take their dogs and they love the exercise too. They never miss a day. Both my sisters are very busy working women and mothers. How do they do it? What keeps them going? It's not optional for them. It's an appointment they keep, like any other appointment or job. Walking gives them energy for all the other important things in their lives. Can you make an appointment to be more physically active? Remember, it's *not* optional. Schedule it like any other activity you have to do.

Throughout history, we've never been this sedentary before; it's a result of living in a land of incredible abundance. We have so many blessings. Yet the very abundance and blessings we enjoy are causing us problems no one could have imagined a few short decades ago.

ARE YOU READY FOR PHYSICAL ACTIVITY?

Are you motivated yet? Well, hold on, Energy Girls! We want this to be a change you make for a lifetime—something you can live with for a very long time—so it's important you follow a few simple guidelines. You'll be happy you did.

For most women, getting up and getting moving is going to provide wonderful benefits. But there are a few women for whom physical activity might be inappropriate, or they should have medical advice first concerning what activities might be best for them. Do you have any of following the conditions?

- Chest pains
- High blood pressure or any heart condition
- Dizziness, or balance problems
- Asthma
- Bone or joint problems
- Diabetes
- Any new, undiagnosed symptom or condition
- Any reason *you know of* that would keep you from engaging in physical activity

If you're pregnant, you also want to check with your doctor before beginning an exercise program, or if you're over the age of 45. Please use common sense. If you have any of the above conditions, the American College of Sports Medicine (ACSM) advises you to seek a medical opinion about the type of exercise that is safe and appropriate for you before you start a physical activity program, and that's the exact recommendation I make.

What is Health-Related Fitness?

There have been many definitions of what physical fitness is, and some of those definitions have changed over the years. Health-related fitness is all about the different elements of fitness that relate to one thing—your good health. Do you have energy as a woman for all your everyday activities and to-do lists? Can you do those activities without getting overly tired? Do you have the energy you need for extra leisure activities, too? Would you have the energy you need to handle any emergency situation you might encounter? Answering yes to those questions is one simple definition of fitness. Whatever definition you use, let me assure you that nothing increases a woman's sense of physical well-being faster than getting on a safe and effective fitness program.

COMPONENTS OF FITNESS

It's a good idea to personalize your health-related fitness program, and you can do that by understanding the basic components of fitness: Aerobic Fitness, Muscular Fitness, Flexibility, and Body Composition.

Aerobic Fitness

Cardiovascular or aerobic fitness helps your body produce more energy. "Cardio" refers to your heart and "vascular" to your blood vessels. The ability of your heart to deliver blood and oxygen to your working muscles during exercise is what cardiovascular (aerobic) exercise is all about. It makes your heart strong. Most women also like the fact that getting in cardiovascular shape helps burn fat the fastest. When you walk briskly, swim, ride a bike, or even climb stairs, you can strengthen your heart and also lower your risk for heart disease.

Muscular Fitness

You need both muscular strength and endurance. Strength refers to how much you can lift safely, and endurance refers to how many times you can lift safely. You need strong muscles to carry groceries, lift a toddler, or do a myriad of everyday tasks. The fastest way to see changes in your body is to combine strength training and aerobic exercise with a low-fat diet. After the age of 20, women lose one pound of muscle every two years if they are inactive. Muscle is active tissue—the more muscle you have, the more calories you burn.

Flexibility

Can you move as freely as you did 10 years ago? As we grow older, we lose flexibility, and most women answer *No*. Flexibility is about how much movement you have around different joints in your body. A safe and effective stretching program can help make sure you keep moving for a lifetime. Do you feel tension in your back, neck, or anywhere in your body? Most women say one of the best benefits they get from stretching is not only increased flexibility but release of tension. Gentle stretching can help you relax.

Body Composition

If health-related fitness is your goal, what you weigh doesn't matter nearly as much as how much of your weight is fat. Too much fat can cause a host of problems for your health, and that's what's most important—not what you look like. As we age, our body fat increases. You can decrease that natural aging process by being on the right kind of health-related fitness program. If you develop more lean tissue and less body fat, it will also change the way you look dramatically.

Energy Girls®
Basic Get-Up-and-Go Fit Facts

- ### When In Doubt, Get Checked Out

Make sure you follow ACSM guidelines that state, "If you have experienced any medical situation requiring a physician's care, or if you have been told to reduce your physical activity for any reason, you should consult your doctor before beginning an exercise program." Before you get up and go, get checked out.

- ### Set Goals

Be realistic. Set simple goals. Create a plan that works for you. That might be as simple as saying, "For the next four weeks, I will go for a walk every other day." If you will commit to any goal you set, you'll experience the added joy of success upon reaching your objective.

Energy for God's Women

• Get Dressed

WORKOUT WEAR - Women are more likely to work out if they feel good about what they work out in. That's not information from a scientific study. It's first-hand, personal experience as a woman. When we're happy about the way we look, we stick with the program. Dress for comfort, but dress for beauty too. Most women feel badly if they've let themselves get out of shape, and staying with a fitness plan is all about motivation. It will definitely motivate you if you have something to get dressed in that's appropriate fitness wear and makes you look good. Make sure your workout clothes are comfortable, breathable and easy-fitting. If you need a reason to go buy something new and beautiful, consider it an investment in your health.

SHOES - Don't scrimp on shoes. Find a comfortable pair of fitness shoes you like, but before you buy them, walk around in them for several minutes to make sure they fit. Is there enough room in the toes? Buy shoes at the end of the day, when your feet are largest. You will get a more accurate fit. Depending on your unique foot shape, one brand of shoe might feel better than another. They are all made a little differently, so don't worry about the brand as much as what works for you—and what feels great. The key point to remember is *comfort*.

• Warm-up and Cool-down

A warm-up prepares your body for more vigorous exercise to come. It's the gradual increase of your heart rate and is an important part of a fitness program. It's also a wonderful time to leave the worries of the day behind and switch gears mentally. A warm-up might be as simple as walking slowly and leisurely for 5 to10 minutes before you start walking briskly, or marching in place. Always cool down at the end of your workout, too, so your heart rate can *gradually* return to normal. The cool-down is the best time to stretch, increase your flexibility, and just relax.

• Energy Girls® Love to Walk

Current national guidelines indicate that, to improve our health and fitness, we need to get physical activity most days of the week, preferably daily for 30 minutes. However, if you're new to all of this, just start walking 5 or 10 minutes a day. The key to success is to start off *very* slowly to prevent injuries, and gradually increase the intensity of your workout. Walking may be the best exercise of all because it's something everyone can do, and no special equipment is needed to get started. Start off with good posture, take long smooth strides, and let your arms swing comfortably at your sides. For fun, you can also get a pedometer and work toward the ultimate goal of walking 10,000 steps a day. You can start at 2,000 steps a day the first week and the second week 3,000 a day, and so on—do whatever is appropriate in your situation. On days when there's bad weather, you can also do something Energy Girls® really love: "mall walk!"

• The Talk Test

Work out at the right intensity by taking the *Talk Test*. It's a simple concept: You must be able to talk while you're exercising. If you can't, slow it down. It's great to be perspiring and invigorated, but if you're huffing and puffing so hard you can't carry on a conversation with a girlfriend, lighten up the intensity until you get enough oxygen so you can talk.

• Be a Strong Woman

Stronger muscles and stronger bones will decrease a woman's risks for osteoporosis. Walking is a weight-bearing activity, but the best way to strengthen your muscles and bones is by lifting dumbbells, or by using strength-training equipment. It's best to consult with a certified health and fitness professional to learn the safest way to add strength training to your personal fitness plan. To get strength training right, get special instruction.

• Too Much, Too Soon

The number one thing beginners do is exercise too intensely, before their bodies can handle it. They get caught up in the excitement of how good they feel, work out too hard, and then suffer an injury or get so sore they can't move the next day. You didn't get out of shape overnight and you don't need to get in shape overnight. Give yourself several weeks to slowly and gradually increase the intensity of your workouts. The key is to start off slowly. That will prevent both injuries and soreness.

• Take Small Steps

There are lots of ways you can include physical activity in your daily routine:

- ✓ Take the stairs, instead of an elevator.
- ✓ Park further away from stores.
- ✓ Take up any hobby or activity that gets you moving.
- ✓ If there's ever an option of driving or walking—choose walking.

• Two Marvelous Motivators

Listen to the Music - Absolutely nothing motivates more than music. Get joyful praise music you can listen to that lifts your heart as you work out. Music is a special gift from God. Most women say it's their favorite motivator to keep them moving, and it's also the number one way to stay inspired.

No pressure - Enjoy the exhilaration of getting your body moving again, without pressure. Work out when you feel the best and, for the first four weeks, think about only one thing—*enjoying* yourself. Get into the habit of working out. Make it a part of your routine. If you focus on having fun and enjoying the process instead of thinking of your workout as being "work," you will condition your mind to look forward to it regularly.

• Expect Setbacks

If you expect a few setbacks, they won't slow you down and discourage you when they come. If you miss a workout or two—or even several—don't use this as an excuse to stop. Just get right back on track and keep moving forward. Also, decide what the best time of day is for you to exercise. Are you a morning person or a night owl? If you know what works best for you, it will help you stick with it.

• The Best Drink on Earth

God made water the best drink on earth. Water is one of the most important components in our bodies. Stay hydrated when you work out. The best way to do that is to drink water before, during and after exercise.

• Don't Make Excuses

"I don't have time." You're right. You will never have time to work out *unless you make it a priority.* We always find time to do the things we want. You have to schedule the time, like any appointment you have to show up for. Decide it's not optional to become more physically active.

"I have no energy. I'm tired." Getting fit is how you will get more energy, remember? After a few weeks on a consistent fitness program, you will have so much more energy that you will be able to do everything more quickly—with energy to spare.

Your Body Type

As you develop your goals, it might help to keep in mind your natural body type as a woman. You don't need to limit yourself, but your fitness goals should be realistic, based on the way God made you.

THE HOURGLASS (Mesomorph) - Women who are broad at the shoulders and hips, narrow at the waist. May look fit without exercise. Medium-to large-boned. Moderate metabolism. With exercise, this body type can drop fat easily and gain definition of muscles.

THE PEAR-SHAPE (Endomorph) - Women who are round, a body with more fat distributed at the hips and thighs. May have a slower metabolism and muscles not as easily defined. Fat will appear to drop off more slowly with exercise. Weight training will help develop muscle definition. Fat will come off hips and thighs last.

THE RULER (Ectomorph) - Women who are long, lean, rectangular. Small-boned. Flat-chested, with slender hips, waist not well-defined. Low body fat compared to other body types. Able to meet the weight chart requirements easily. Faster metabolism naturally.

As a woman, you may be one type or most likely a combination of body types, and that's the way God made you. You don't have the ability to change your body type, but you do have the ability to be the best you can be for the body type you have. God did not make all women to look alike—Hollywood to the contrary. You can look at creation and see the wonderful variety in everything God made. He made women in different colors, shapes, and sizes. And he made you exactly the way he wants you.

Seasons in a Woman's Life

Women experience many seasons. Becoming mothers, nurturing others, experiencing childbirth, dramatic hormonal changes and illnesses—all can be a part of the seasons of a woman's life. We need to do the best we can in each special season. There are times when simply moving forward can be challenging.

Energy Girls® Fact!

Becoming mothers, nurturing others, experiencing childbirth, dramatic hormonal changes and illnesses—all can be a part of the seasons of a woman's life.

My dear friend and elderly neighbor, Muriel, first had one stroke and then another. She was a very strong woman and always tried to be active, even at age 89. After her second stroke, the big moment came when she could finally go outside for a walk. She was determined to simply walk to the mailbox, albeit very slowly with me cheering her on. For that season and stage in her life, she wasn't just doing well—she was phenomenal.

My dearest friend and professional colleague, Tina, had a rough time when she had her second baby. Her sweet little boy had to stay in the hospital several extra weeks. He finally came home with a heart monitor, and she came home with an infection that contributed to throwing her into a tailspin with a true-blue post-partum depression. When I saw her then, she could barely function. I said, "Tina, girl, we're getting you some help!" She was off to the doctor's where she got just the care she needed, and in very little time she was her old self again. It was an important time because God used it to teach her things in the midst of this trial. However, during that time, the last thing she could think about was extra physical activity—or any physical activity—but it was just for a *season*.

When I was a very young woman, I battled cancer and had several surgeries. In the midst of that battle, I needed help just to walk. I couldn't even get to the kitchen without family, good girlfriends, and an all-out effort. Up to that point, I had always been an energetic, strong woman, and it was quite a switch. With God's grace, I did the best I could. After repeated surgeries and procedures, I knew my body was not going to be what it once was. It was a new season. As I kept my eyes on Jesus, I learned *"that God causes everything to work together for the good of those who love God and are called according to his purpose for them"* Romans 8: 28 (NLT). I'm very glad that doesn't say, "almost all things work for good" or "most things work for good." It says, ALL things work for good. And that's true for you, too, as God's woman, no matter what season of life you're in now.

Are you weary from being a mother 24/7? Are you someone's constant caregiver and feel like you have nothing left to give? What setbacks have you had? What season are you in? Do you feel physically weak? If so, here's good news. "My grace is all you need. My power works best in weakness." So now I am glad to boast about my weaknesses, so that the power of Christ can work through me" 2 Corinthians 12:9 (NLT).

I thank God for what I went through because it enabled me to understand physical weakness, to know how to comfort others, and to know where my true strength lies—in Jesus alone. You need to do the best you can now, in this particular season of your life, and trust God with the rest. We need to be good stewards of the bodies God has given us, but that doesn't mean we're perfect. Whew! What a relief. Energy Girls, get moving any way you can—it's the fastest way to increase your energy level and promote your health.

THE POWER OF FOOD

God wants you to enjoy food. He gave you taste buds and created an amazing variety of foods for you to eat. In fact, he didn't just give you a few taste buds, he gave you around 10,000. You can taste sweet, sour, salty, bitter and savory. He did that so you could *enjoy* eating.

Do you ever wonder what it was like when the Lord first created the earth? On that day when he placed both man and woman in the Garden? Sometimes I think about it, but I'm sure the beauty of it is beyond our imagining. Not only were man and woman perfect, the food was, too. Everything in the beginning was without spot or blemish.

> **God spoke: "Earth, green up! Grow all varieties of seed-bearing plants, every sort of fruit-bearing tree." And there it was. Earth produced green seed-bearing plants, all varieties, and fruit-bearing trees of all sorts. God saw that it was good.**
>
> Genesis 1:11-12 (MSG)

There were no diets and no one was worrying about eating too much or too little. No workouts were needed because there were no health problems, and everyone had more than enough energy. In heaven, we will never have health concerns again.

I'm grateful and in awe of everything the Lord created. It says clearly in scripture when you look at creation, you can see the hand of God at work. "Through everything God made, they can clearly see his invisible qualities" Romans 1:20b (NLT).

I don't usually shop at night, but recently I had to get something very late at our large local grocery store. I was the only one in the big produce section. As I looked around at the dazzling display, it was as if I were seeing things for the very first time. I could only marvel at the rainbow of colors and the variety of fruits and vegetables that God made. The lush fruits and vegetables in the garden must have been beyond anything we can comprehend, and how much Adam and Eve must have enjoyed it all. No diets for them! Not a worry in the world about eating too much or about not having enough to eat.

> Then God said, "Look! I have given you every seed-bearing plant throughout the earth and all the fruit trees for your food.
>
> Genesis 1:29 (NLT)

How much power does food have in your life? Of course, food has no power at all—only the power we give it. Women tend to give far too *much* power to food and their weight. And many women suffer pain and frustration over this issue. Most women I know spend a lot of time worrying about food and what they should or shouldn't eat. We are the nurturers and caretakers of our families, so we tend to be around food a lot too, preparing meals and serving others. Women don't have a normal relationship to food, and I don't think the men in our lives completely understand the issue. One day, my husband finally confirmed this for me. I asked him if he and the other men he knew had a normal relationship with food, and he said, "I've never *once* thought about having a relationship with food!" Ah, women and food—the never-ending relationship struggle.

I've seen women completely panic when they have to get on a scale. Many years ago, I directed a number of health screening fairs for corporations with the goal of trying to reduce employee

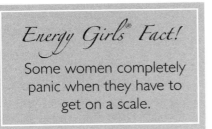

Energy Girls® Fact!

Some women completely panic when they have to get on a scale.

health risks and health care costs. At the health screenings, we took weight, height, and basic body composition measurements. After thousands of assessments, I will tell you in a nutshell what I observed.

Women are phobic about their weight, and do you know what men have a huge issue with? Their *height*. Man after man simply had to exaggerate their height or wouldn't believe what I told them. I might say, "You're 5' 11", and they would say emphatically, "No, I'm not, I'm 6 feet tall!"

Women, on the other hand, would panic when we asked them to weigh-in. They would sometimes cover their eyes—or simply refuse to get on the scale. Those that did get on it would often look completely devastated, crushed, or depressed, and explain that it was "that time of month," or they were bloated, or they had just gained five pounds and they were *really* going to lose the weight. The weigh-ins didn't last long. The scales stood empty. Every woman knows what I'm talking about—weight is an issue. If you're one of the very few women who do not know what I'm talking about because you have never, ever had to worry about your weight, I have something to say to you: "It's not fair!" Now, for the rest of us—here's crucial information.

SUPER SIZE!

Today, the diet industry is a $35 billion business. Even with all the diets, 61 percent of adults in the U.S. are still overweight, and the problem continues to grow. We live in a sedentary society, we have

Energy for God's Wome

more food choices than ever before, we eat on the go, and we're exposed to marketing and advertising encouraging us to "Super Size!" The movie of the same name made clear America's love with fast food—and big portions.

We are a nation of choices. Why not make choices that will help you live a healthier lifestyle? Steven Anderson, president of the National Restaurant Association, said, "Blaming the food industry for obesity among Americans is really swallowing a simplistic notion." In a way, he's right. Americans spend more than $110 billion on fast food. And each dollar is about someone making a choice and a selection about what they want to eat. In America, we daily choose to eat 2,400,000 Burger King Whoppers and 1,900,000 Krispy Kreme glazed doughnuts. That's a lot of fat and calories.

Only 19 percent of Americans feel free from worrying about weight loss and gain, and studies show that 95 percent of all those who diet gain the weight back. Did you know that health and fitness centers actually count on a very high attrition rate to stay in business? They know most people have a hard time sticking with their diet and exercise program, and that enables them to sell many more memberships than they can accommodate. They are aware that after a few weeks, most of the people won't show up.

It would indeed be wonderful if we didn't have to worry about our weight or this issue. If only we could enjoy our food in a completely normal way. Let it have its proper place of importance—not too little and not too much. That would mean we would eat when we're hungry, and we would stop when we're full, naturally. We would enjoy what we ate, be satisfied and thank God for his provision. Then we would know when it was time to eat again because our hunger mechanism would give us the signal, just the way God intended. We wouldn't be panicked and guilt-ridden around food. We wouldn't feel out of control around food either—or eat too much. We would simply enjoy what we ate with thanksgiving.

> ## Energy Girls® Fact!
>
> Women eat for a lot of reasons. We're hungry, bored, depressed, worried, stressed, need comfort, want to be polite, or just because the food is there.

Women eat for a lot of reasons. We're hungry, bored, depressed, worried, stressed, need comfort, want to be polite, or just because the food is there. God gave us a hunger mechanism so we would know when to eat, and so we could thoroughly enjoy our food and also be satisfied. The problem is that most of us don't know what normal eating is anymore. We've been "dieted out"—starved up and down, on diets, off diets, and filled with so much guilt about eating too much fat or too many calories that we've thrown our own "full" mechanism out of whack. The last thing you need to hear about is another diet, and that's a good thing because diets don't work.

What does work?

Pray and ask for God's guidance, so you can make healthy choices based on your needs and God's provision. If you make the right choices every day, over time you will get the results you want and you'll keep you and your family healthy in the process. If you maintain an active lifestyle through a health-related fitness program, that will give you the very best energy results, plus it will speed up your metabolism and help you burn both calories and body fat. You need to think "big picture." You need to adopt a healthier lifestyle for the rest of your life.

Studies show that a good diet, plus the right kind of exercise, is the number one way to keep weight off and increase your energy. All it takes are simple changes and easy choices. Take the pressure off. You can't fail with God on your side—and if you fall or don't think you can change, think again; because, with God, "all things are possible." Either God cares about all the little issues in our life, including what we eat, or he doesn't. I believe he cares. If you combine eating right with increasing your physical activity, you will get the very best results. Your health will improve and you will have more energy than you ever thought possible.

Energy Girls® Eat for Health - Basic Top Tips

EAT YOUR FRUITS AND VEGGIES

God made fantastic fruits and veggies to give your body the vitamins, minerals, and fiber you need to do your best. Better yet, almost all of them are low in fat and calories. Eating more fruits and vegetables may even protect

> *Energy Girls® Fact!*
> God made fantastic fruits and veggies to give your body the vitamins, minerals, and fiber you need to do your best.

you from many chronic diseases. Most come in their own "nature" package, ready to pop in your purse or your little one's lunch bag. Some studies show that only 10 percent of Americans eat enough of these beautiful, colorful gifts—packaged by God. As a woman, you need more fruits and veggies, and so do your loved ones.

Top Tips - How to Do It

- Look for color at the produce section and try to eat a *rainbow* of colors. Dark green leafy lettuce. Broccoli. Red peppers. Carrots. Blueberries. Oranges. Apples. More colors in fruits and vegetables mean a variety of nutrients.
- Buy fruits and vegetables in season for better savings and quality.
- Use a microwave to prepare frozen vegetables, so they're ready in a flash.
- Eat a piece of fruit every day, as a mid-afternoon snack.
- Make a simple, quick fruit salad by chopping up an apple, adding a few chopped nuts, and low-fat yogurt.
- Make sure your fruit juice choices are 100% juice. If you're watching calories, limit yourself to 1 Cup (8oz) a day because you can easily "drink" too many calories in a short period of time. Fresh fruit is an excellent, healthy option.

FAST FAT FACTS

Fat gives foods great taste and flavor, which is the reason we like it so much. But fat is very high in calories, as every woman knows. We eat too much fat, especially too much "saturated" fat, which is bad for our hearts. Saturated fat is hard at room temperature and it comes mostly from animal sources; but watch out for coconut and palm oils, too, since they are also considered saturated. Too much saturated fat can increase your risk for heart disease.

We also eat too much "trans" fat. That's a type of fat that takes liquid oils and turns them into solid fats by a process called "hydrogenation." Trans fat is found in vegetable shortening and hard margarine, in many processed snack foods, baked goods of all kinds, and, of course, in many fried foods. Like saturated fat, trans fat is bad news. It tends to raise bad LDL cholesterol, lower one's good HDL cholesterol, and it can also increase our risk for heart disease. According to the FDA, the average American eats about 4.7 pounds of trans fats each year. Because trans fats extend the shelf life of foods and are in so many products today, a new law now requires they be listed on food labels. (For the first time *ever*, a Board of Health has actually banned all trans fats in restaurants in New York City.) Monounsaturated fats are the good guys in the world of fats and they can be found in things like olive and canola oils. Polyunsaturated fats are mostly from plants too—also good guys. They can be found in nuts and oils that are made from soybeans, corn, and sunflowers. The bottom line is that you and your family need to eat less fat overall, and especially less "bad" fats.

> *Energy Girls® Fact!*
> According to the FDA, the average American eats about 4.7 pounds of trans fats each year.

Top Tips - How to Do It

- Remove visible fat from beef and poultry or simply remove the skin completely from chicken.
- Make small changes. For example, replace mayonnaise that's high in fat with mustard that is virtually fat-free.

- Pack healthy low-fat snacks and, if you visit fast-food restaurants, check out the menu and pick low-fat items. Even a plain hamburger can be a good choice, compared to a "Double Whopper with Cheese" at 990 calories and 64 grams of total fat.
- If you love specialty coffee drinks, make sure when you order lattes or cappuccinos that you say, "Skim, please."
- Read labels and learn to understand them. Know what kind of fats you are currently eating and watch out for hidden fats in processed snack foods.

THE "WHOLE" IN WHOLE GRAINS

Whole grains add important fiber, vitamins and minerals to your diet. Very few Americans eat enough of them. Whole-grain foods have all the good stuff left in the grain, just the way God intended. Refined grains, like white flour, "refine" or remove the healthiest part of the grain—the bran and the germ. That's the part that has most of the nutrients. You have to be very wise when you read food labels. It can be tricky. Companies often try to make you think their products are whole grain, even if they're not. If you want to buy whole grain bread, see if the *first* ingredient on the label says "whole wheat" or "100% whole wheat." The key is the word "whole." The words "wheat flour" and "enriched flour" are *not* whole grain. To meet the US Dietary guidelines, make at least one-half of *all* the grains you eat in a full day "whole." You can also eat other whole grains like corn, barley, oats, or brown rice. One study showed that women who ate more whole grains daily *weighed less*. Women who eat whole grains

Energy Girls® Fact!

Whole-grain foods have all the good stuff left in the grain, just the way God intended.

Energy for God's Wom

have decreased hunger and may also reduce health risks for many diseases. Another study at the University of Minnesota showed that older women in Iowa who ate whole grains over 11 years outlived women who ate "refined" grains.

Top Tips - How to Do It

- Simply replace one "refined" food product you normally eat with one whole-grain product.
- Make oatmeal, a breakfast tradition—"rolled" oats are best. Or try a whole-grain, ready-to-eat cold cereal and top it off with fresh fruit.
- Popcorn is a healthy whole grain—without the butter!
- Substitute one-half of any recipe that uses white flour with "whole wheat" flour.
- Add brown rice or another whole grain to soups or casseroles.
- Enjoy baked corn tortilla chips. They're a delicious whole grain snack and, with salsa, almost fat-free.

DAIRY AND CALCIUM FOR STRONG BONES

Women need strong bones. Our bones weaken as we age, and our risks for developing osteoporosis increase. One in two women will have an osteoporosis-related fracture in her lifetime. Calcium gives us the nutrients we need for strong bone health. Of course, you also need to add the right amount of weight-bearing exercises, in a health-related fitness program, to keep your bones strong. New studies show that dairy products not only provide needed calcium,

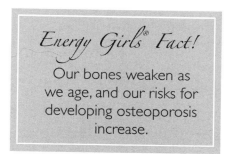

Energy Girls® Fact!
Our bones weaken as we age, and our risks for developing osteoporosis increase.

they might also lower blood pressure. Make sure to choose low-fat or nonfat dairy items, always the best choice. Another study showed that when adults and children increased the dairy and calcium in their diets, they had less of a tendency to become overweight. Don't forget, calcium can also be found in some vegetables, like collard and turnip greens, broccoli and spinach. It's also found in sardines and canned salmon with bones. You can also choose calcium fortified cereals, juices and breads. However you get the right amount of calcium, just make sure you do it. It's very important for a woman's health.

Top Tips - How to Do It

- Choose low-fat or fat-free dairy products, like skim milk and low-fat yogurt.
- Use low-fat plain yogurt in place of mayonnaise or sour cream in dips for vegetables.
- In a blender, put skim milk or powdered milk, fresh frozen fruit, and a sweetener of your choice, for a delicious fruit smoothie.
- Get extra calcium by adding low-fat or nonfat milk to soups.
- Top a whole grain or multi-grain English muffin with melted low-fat cheese, like mozzarella.
- Drink calcium-fortified orange juice.
- For a delicious snack choose apple slices and a few cubes of low-fat cheese.

THINK LEAN FOR PROTEIN

Your body uses protein to repair body tissues including organs, skin, muscles, bones and teeth. Protein helps produce red blood cells, hormones and helps your immune system do its job. Protein provides the basic building blocks of the human body. Most Americans get more than enough protein, but new information shows something very interesting. In a recent study, participants who added a little

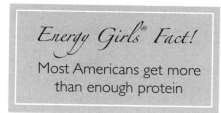

extra lean protein to breakfast felt fuller, more satisfied, and less hungry for the next four hours. Most people in the U.S. eat a great deal of animal protein and since that's usually high in saturated fat, it's best for heart health to choose lean meats, poultry, fish, beans, and nuts. If you think lean, you will also reduce your calories, and if you add just the right amount of protein at breakfast, you may help reduce hunger pangs too.

Top Tips - How to Do It

- If you buy ground beef, choose extra lean (Look for at least 90 percent lean).
- Poultry choices are best when they're skinless.
- Think broil, bake, and grill—*not* fried.
- Eat more fish. Frozen is easier to find and usually less expensive.
- Buy water packed tuna and make tuna salad with low-fat yogurt.
- Nuts, a great protein source can be added as a garnish or topping to oatmeal, cold cereals, salads, quick breads, and sandwiches. Remember, they're high in fat, so add sparingly.
- Enjoy beans, another great protein. Use "hummus" dip—made from garbanzo beans—and serve with cut-up vegetables.

Fill Your Grocery Cart with the All the Right Stuff

It's easy to start eating for health and energy. When you go grocery shopping, before you start loading your grocery cart up, remember:

- ✓ Choose more fruits, vegetables, whole grains, and fat-free or low-fat dairy products.
- ✓ Choose proteins such as lean meats, poultry, fish, beans, eggs, or nuts.
- ✓ Read labels and select foods with less fats, trans fats, cholesterol, salt and sugars.

Bonus tips:

- ★ Always go to the grocery store with a list to avoid impulse buying.
- ★ Shop the perimeter of the grocery store. It's there you will find whole foods, fruits, vegetables, low-fat dairy products, and lean meats.
- ★ Don't go grocery shopping on an empty stomach. Make sure you eat something before you go, so you're not tempted to buy all the irresistible goodies.

ENERGY GIRLS®' RULES FOR EATING - SIMPLE AS 1, 2, 3!

Three simple rules to help you make changes *now*:

SIMPLE RULE #1 - KNOW WHAT YOU SHOULD EAT.
Do you understand the basics of what you should eat? Educate yourself. To make the right choices you need to know the basic facts. Don't be a mindless eater. Know what you *should* eat. The more you know, the better choices you will make.

SIMPLE RULE #2 - ASSESS HOW YOU REALLY EAT.

Assess what you *really* eat. For the next 48 hours, write down your food choices. Don't change anything. Just write it down, *when you eat it*. You won't remember otherwise. Then compare it with what you should be eating.

SIMPLE RULE #3 - CHANGE WHAT YOU DO EAT.

If you know what you should eat, and you've assessed what you actually eat—what's the difference between the two? Once you answer this question, you will know the very first steps you need to take, so you can eat for health and energy. It's time to *change* what you do eat. And the best time to start doing that is *right now*.

When All Else Fails

Do you feel like you've struggled with the issue of food and your weight for so long that there's no hope for you? Have you prayed and prayed? *Then God has heard your cry.* Ask him to teach you something in the midst of your struggle. Don't look at things the way the world does—look at things as God's woman.

Perhaps you could have someone else pray with you, try a new approach to modify your eating habits, or see your physician to see if there might be a physical reason why you can't experience victory. Throughout a woman's life, there are many reasons why she might gain or lose weight. Child-bearing and hormonal changes through the years make it especially challenging, and so does the fact that women naturally carry more body fat than men. It's just the way God designed us.

There's even a chance you're not ready to make the commitment needed. Do you really want to change? Sometimes we say we want to change, but we're only kidding ourselves. We're not fooling God. He knows our every thought and sees our hearts.

It can be hard to change, and sometimes it's uncomfortable. All really good things take work and effort. You can even pray and ask God to help you to *want to change*—-to give you the desire to do what it takes, and to give you the strength. It doesn't matter how you feel, God is waiting to hear from you. Make a few simple changes, pray, and see what good things begin to happen. Let food take its proper place in your life, and experience the freedom of having a normal relationship with food.

If you feel you've been in bondage to the power of food, know that Jesus wants to set you free. You were created to be God's woman, to serve him with your whole heart, soul, and mind. Remember that food was created to nourish your body, not to cause you guilt and pain. Eat for health and for energy. Let God take over in every area of your life and ask him to make you a wise woman when it comes to dealing with food.

Step 5: Your Magnificent Mission

When it's all been said and done
There is just one thing that matters
Did I do my best to live for Truth
Did I live my life for You

Jim Cowan

*F*aint streaks of light began to appear in the sky as I
watched the sun come up from the top floor of my
hotel room. I was scheduled to speak at a convention and
was up early, reading and praying. My husband was still
fast asleep. He's a night owl and I'm a morning person.
I'm always up by 5:00 a.m.—without an alarm. When I
first looked out the window, it was totally dark. But then,
the faintest rays of morning light started to appear. As
always, it was *amazing*.

The Lord's mercies are new every morning. The
most obvious sign is the way he lifts the darkness away
in a few seconds with his light. I watched as it got lighter
and lighter until I could finally see clearly. Far off in
the distance were mountains. Right below me, I could
see freeways and speeding cars—*thousands* of them.
They were the loopy kind of freeways, with overpasses,

underpasses, and figure-eights. Cars were going up and down, over each other, and around the bend—all driving as fast as they could to their various destinations.

From the top floor, as I was looking down at the cars and vehicles speeding below me—each one racing along—I could only guess who the drivers were. I couldn't see them. *Where were they going?* I wondered. *To an office, back home from the night shift, perhaps returning from a hospital visit, or were moms driving their kids to school?* The Lord knew where every single person had been, where they were going, and their final destination. All of a sudden I started thinking about how brief life is. It occurred to me that in 100 years every person—every single one—in all the vehicles racing along, would be gone.

Only one thing really matters.

We're so busy. We're in such a hurry. We feel everything we do is so important and everything that can be done must be done—by us. But women can't do it all. There is only one way to find your true magnificent mission, and that's by having a relationship with the one who created you. That's actually why you were created, to have a relationship and be in fellowship with God—forever and ever.

Jesus, the one and only.

Your Creator. Your Redeemer. Your Deliverer. Your Rock. Your Healer. Your Savior. Your Righteousness. The First and the Last.

To fulfill your magnificent mission you absolutely, positively have to be right with God first. Are you God's woman *completely*? Is there anything in your life you're holding on to, or something you're not ready to let go of? God wants all of you. He wants to give you his peace. To receive God's rest and peace you have to give him only one thing—*your heart*.

Energy for God's Wome

If you haven't done that before, or if you need to do it again, don't hesitate. I love that God makes it so simple. You can talk to him anytime. Turn your heart to him no matter where you are—or where you have been. *You can even do it right now.*

There's Always Hope

Life here can be difficult, challenging, draining, and sometimes filled with heartbreak and disappointment. With God on your side, the difference is that everything in your day can take on special, divine significance. *That's energizing.* When you give your life to Christ, you receive a magnificent mission. Even the troubles in your day will be used to make you a stronger woman of God. If you remember that, it will help you keep your daily trials in perspective. Then you will be filled with hope no matter what happens—and nothing gives energy and joy like a heart filled with hope. One study of women aged 24 to 35 revealed that 51 percent of them felt bored or hopeless when they thought about the future. Clearly, many women need hope. Our God is *the* God of hope, and we need to keep our eyes on him.

> **And so Lord, where do I put my hope? My only hope is in you.**
>
> Psalm 39:7 (NLT)

Have a Clear Vision

If you know your magnificent mission—your relationship to God—you also need to remember you're not living for yourself anymore, you're living for Christ. How does that change your motives? How do you live as a woman of God and make the *right* decisions about where and how to spend your daily time and energy? Women are tired, drained and exhausted, and we keep trying to do it all; but as women of faith, aren't we supposed to be living differently? You need to have a clear vision. Without one, you will end up lost. It's been said, "If you don't know where you're going, any road will lead you there." You don't want to waste energy all day long, trying to figure out where you're going.

From the time I was a little girl, I've had vision problems. I've always had to wear glasses. Without my glasses everything is fuzzy and out of focus. When I go to bed, if I don't carefully put my glasses *exactly* where they're supposed to be, when I wake up in the morning I can't see well enough to find them. But the minute I put my glasses on (or contacts in)—Wow! I can see everything. It fills me with confidence and I step right out and do what needs to be done. I have a clear sense of direction. When you have clear vision, it will make everything you do easier and it will take less energy. That's the way you should feel when you put on your spiritual glasses, and you do that by focusing on the number one relationship in your life. God must come first.

When you wake up in the morning, you need to armor yourself spiritually. For you, that might mean getting up early for quiet time and reading the Word of God, or getting on your knees to pray as soon as you get out of bed, or even listening to praise music as you're getting ready for work. Your schedule and situation are unique and I don't know what works for you, but whatever it takes, stay focused and prayerful at the start of each new day. If you do that first, you will be ready, trusting in God and seeing clearly, no matter what happens. As God's woman, you want to make loving responses and wise decisions, knowing you're investing your time and energy on your real mission. Make sure you put on your spiritual glasses every morning, so you know where you're going.

If people can't see what God is doing, they stumble all over themselves; but when they attend to what he reveals, they are most blessed.

Proverbs 29:18 (MSG)

Be the Best Woman

To have a clear sense of purpose all day, you need to thoughtfully and prayerfully think ahead of time about your priorities. Take charge of everything you can and have a plan. That means planning but also being flexible, in case the unexpected happens. Be the best woman of God you can be in every hour, in every situation. If that's being a wife, be the best wife you can be. If that's being a single woman, be the best single woman you can be. If that's being a mother, be the best mother you can be. If that's being an employee, be the best employee you can be. Let God direct your steps, and he will give you the energy you need for what he's called you to do. Make a decision to seek him in every situation. Then, instead of wasting energy fretting, fuming, and being frazzled when things "go wrong," you can, by faith, trust that God is working all things together for your good. You will be living out your magnificent mission and you will be on an exciting spiritual adventure with God.

> *Show me the path where I should walk, O LORD; point out the right road for me to follow.*
>
> Psalm 25:4 (NLT)

> *Seek his will in all that you do, and he will direct your paths.*
>
> Proverbs 3:6 (NLT)

Your Magnificent Mission List

You also need clear vision, so you will know what God's priorities are for your life, hour by hour. You can't do it all and sometimes you need to say *Yes* with your time and energy but sometimes you need to say *No*. Contrary to how most women live, you can't *always* say *Yes*. We are nurturers and relationship-oriented and we don't like saying no to anyone when we're asked to help. And surely there are many times that we need to help and serve, whether we're tired or not, gifted or not, or have time or not. But there are also definitely times we need to say *No*, because if we don't, we won't have the time and energy to do the things God has called us to do. How do you know the difference? You create a Magnificent Mission List.

To create a Magnificent Mission List you need to know, without doubt, that you want whatever God wants for your life. That will help you clearly hear what he is saying. Knowing you have totally given your life to Christ is the key, because then you will begin to learn how he oftentimes puts his desires in your heart.

> *Take delight in the Lord, and he will give you your heart's desires. Commit everything you do to the Lord. Trust him, and he will help you.*
>
> Psalm 37: 4-5 (NLT)

> *You will find him if you look for him with all your heart and with all your soul.*
>
> Deuteronomy 4:29 (NLT)

Look into your heart. What is God saying to you? Sometimes God speaks quietly in my heart. It's beyond words. Sometimes I have an idea that I can't let go of, or I feel great passion and enthusiasm about something I feel I must do. I've learned over time, that's one of the ways the Lord speaks to me. I'm also careful to submit my ideas and plans to the people God has put in my life. In my case, that's my husband, my dearest godly girlfriends (the Energy Girls!) and other mature people I trust. I also make sure everything lines up with scripture.

God can speak to us in several ways: Through the scriptures, his written Word, through circumstances, through other people, and by impressing our hearts and minds directly by the power of the Holy Spirit. The more you obey him, the more clearly you will hear him.

To create your magnificent mission list you need to be quiet, think, and pray. See if you can go on a mini-retreat or take half a Saturday and get away. If you can't get away, go off to a corner in your own house, to the library, or even sit in your car—in a quiet, safe place. Just do what it takes. You're a unique woman. I don't know your situation but God does, so do whatever works for *you*. Get out a clean piece of paper and write at the top "**My Magnificent Mission**," then simply write down what you *know* are your top three priorities in life. These are the things, without a doubt, you should be spending your time and energy on.

My Top Three Priorities

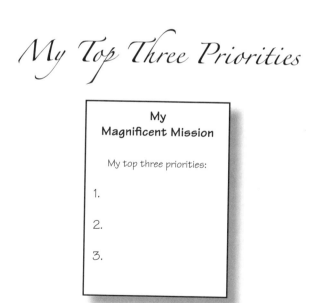

My
Magnificent Mission

My top three priorities:

1.

2.

3.

Your List of Things to Do

After you've done that, on another blank piece of paper write down everything you do and everything you're involved in, daily and weekly. Make a list that will show you—at a glance—all your responsibilities, your projects, things you belong to, extracurricular activities, *every single thing that takes your time and energy during the day.* Your list might go on and on, or it might be quite short. Either way is fine. There's no right or wrong way to do this. Just pray for God's insights as you write.

List of all the things I do:

Roles I have, hats I wear, my daily to-do list. Everything that takes my time and energy. . . .

1.	6.
2.	7.
3.	8.
4.	9.
5.	10.
	To be cont. . .

Once you've completed both lists, compare them. *How much time and energy are you spending on things that have nothing to do with your God-given priorities?* We are being bombarded constantly with every conceivable idea of what we could and should be doing with our time and energy. Never before in history have women had these many options and choices. But most of the ideas and options are not God's way, and you're God's woman, remember? Are you drained every day because you're simply trying to do *too* much?

> **If you want to know what God wants you to do—ask him, and he will gladly tell you.**
>
> James 1:5a (NLT)

Look at your two lists and compare them closely again. Write down two simple things you can do, *two action steps* that will enable you to spend more time and energy on your real priorities.

**My
Magnificent Mission**

Two Action Steps
I will take so I can
spend time on my real
priorities.

1. _____

2. _____

My friend and colleague, Tina, and I do this exercise when we need to refocus on God's priorities for our lives. Just recently, after doing this exercise together, she told me that she decided to begin a structured Bible study in the morning. She wants to be more focused on God when she starts her day. She's also going to stop teaching a fitness class for women at the local Y. She loves teaching the class, but for now, for this season in her life, it doesn't fit into her other, more important, God-given priorities—being a wife and mother of three little ones. And it's those priorities that need her time and energy.

Is your life too complicated? Sometimes simpler is better. What can you simplify? Granted, this is a challenge because most of us are locked in to our current routines and schedules, as crazy as they might be—*they're ours*—and we don't want to change a thing. It will take time to stop and develop a plan to simplify any area of your life. But if you take that time now, it will actually make things easier for you. It will take you less energy to do the basics and give you more energy for other things in your life. Try to create a simpler system for grocery shopping, doing laundry, household cleaning, or running errands. What specific area of your life can you order and simplify so you will have more time for your real mission? Take one more piece of paper and write down what two action steps you can take to *simplify* your life.

```
┌─────────────────────────────┐
│            My               │
│    Magnificent Mission      │
│                             │
│    Two Action Steps I will  │
│    take to simplify my life.│
│                             │
│    1. _____  │
│                             │
│                             │
│    2. _____  │
│                             │
└─────────────────────────────┘
```

Live Your Mission

Don't Waste Time and Energy - Top Tips!

- **Write Out a "Daily Mission List."**
  Women who accomplish big things make lists and write things down. A list will simply help you stay focused on what's most important. It's like getting directions when you're driving somewhere, instead of guessing where you're going. If you write down a simple list in the morning of what you want to accomplish, you can keep it as a reminder all day long, so you stay *on* mission.

- **Remember God's Faithfulness.**

  When you lose sight of your mission and you feel discouraged, call another Energy Girl, or a friend who can be a "Hope Coach." Recount God's faithfulness in your lives. Scripture tells us to do that. You will be filled with hope and encouragement if you stop to remember God's faithfulness in the past.

- **Do a Motivation Check.**

  Your magnificent mission is about living for Christ—not for yourself. You want to use your amazing gifts, have energizing relationships, declutter your life, and take care of your body so you can do your best for God—not so you can receive the applause and approval of men and women. Don't waste time being a "people pleaser"; instead, focus on pleasing God.

- **Don't Just React, Remain Calm.**

  When your day starts getting very busy and you feel like a tornado hit, *don't* react to the chaos around you. The quickest way to waste energy and time is to lose your focus and purpose in the midst of a difficult situation. Decide ahead of time that whenever your daily tornados hit, you will remain calm and *pray*.

- **Be Ready to Swim Upstream.**

  If you have decided to live out your Magnificent Mission with God, not everyone is going to like it. The scriptures promise that. The world's going one way; you're going another. Sometimes that might mean you may feel like you're swimming upstream. *Keep swimming!* Be a righteous woman and remember other Energy Girls® are swimming right beside you.

Don't Give Up - God is with You

Do you have a dream in your heart? Something you believe God has called you to do? Has he given you a vision for something, but you've been waiting so long that you've begun to doubt you ever heard from God? Don't grow weary. The tiniest acorn grows into the strongest tree in the world, the mighty oak—and it's planted and watered by God. The tree takes years to grow, but in time its beautiful limbs finally reach toward the sky. Strong women of God are not made overnight, and it might take time, but wait and see what God does. Even now, he might be working in ways you can only imagine to bring to fruition the very dream he's placed in your heart.

> *Energy Girls® Tip*
>
> Don't give up. God sees what you are doing. You may not see it now, but the Lord has promised that what you offer for love and for truth—for him—will stand the test of time.

Have you ever longed to make a difference in someone's life? Perhaps you've tried to help your spouse, children, friend, family member, someone at church, or at work. Maybe you're a teacher trying to inspire young hearts and minds with God's truth. When you've given so much of yourself—all you have to give—have you ever become weary and wondered, *Did I make a difference? Did I touch anyone's life or change it in any way? Was what I did forgotten?* I can tell you, whatever you offer in love will never be forgotten by God. You must share the gifts God has given you. Don't give up. God sees what you are doing. You may not see it now, but the Lord has promised that what you offer for love and for truth—for him—will

> *Energy Girls® Question*
>
> Have you ever longed to make a difference in someone's life?

stand the test of time. Offer what he gives you, and then trust and *believe* him.

You may have already touched many more lives than you know—even though you haven't seen the fruit of all your efforts, yet. Sometimes God does let us see, and how joyful it is when he does that. But this is a walk of faith, and faith means we walk and trust here on earth, even though we can't see it all *right now*. This is the only place we will need faith, because one day in heaven we will see everything clearly. We won't need faith then.

> *Energy Girls® Tip*
> This is a walk of faith, and faith means we walk and trust here on earth, even though we can't see it all *right now*.

Let God use your gifts and talents for his purposes, and offer your life to him completely. Let love rule in all your relationships. Live in a way that will allow you to simplify your life enough to give you the energy you need for what matters most, and for what God has called you to do. Be a good steward, as best you can, of your body—his temple. And remember, there's no condemnation. Your heavenly Father wants to encourage you and he accepts with love what you offer him, because he looks at your heart.

I'm praying for you. And I trust you will have many stories of faith to tell one day. Stories of God's great faithfulness, just like the story I want to tell you now. *A short story near and dear to my heart that I wrote years ago.* It's about my life and a little song with wings—and how I met the wonderful man I married…

God's Great Purposes...

*The Lord will fulfill his
purpose for me.*

Psalm 138:8 (NIV)

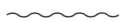

The Butterfly Song Story

The Little Song with Wings

"That new guy is really cute," my girlfriend whispered. "Who is he?" Sarah and I glanced at the young man standing at the front of the church. "That's Brian, he just moved here from Colorado," I answered for the tenth time that day. It seemed all the single women were asking the *same* question. They were obviously excited about our church's new worship leader. I was, too. Although it was many years ago, I can still picture the handsome young man, tall and lean, standing there with a guitar slung over his shoulder.

We first met at Bible study. He played the guitar and I prepared hot cinnamon rolls and drinks for coffee hour after the study. The wafting aroma of those freshly baked sweet rolls always made heads turn, but Brian seemed especially interested. I later discovered that cinnamon rolls hot out of the oven were his favorite. During our long conversations, his good looks and talent were charming, but I had never known a young man who loved God so intensely. I was impressed with his heart.

"Do you know," Brian asked me one day, "how far butterflies can fly on their fragile wings?" Actually, I had never thought about that. "Do you know," he continued, "that elephants can swim in deep water and use their trunks as snorkels?" I had definitely never thought about *that*. God had given Brian a gift to see things in a way that was funny, unique, and full of wonder. And it was contagious! Before long, I was also thanking the Lord for creating Monarch butterflies that can migrate 3,000 miles, and for snorkeling elephants that can swim in deep water. Brian even had me thinking that a crocodile *smiles* when it opens its mouth and shows its big, abundant teeth. I couldn't believe it—I was *actually* thanking the Lord for a smiling crocodile.

As Brian and I became friends, I learned that he and his six sisters had grown up near the woods and, as a child, he spent hours exploring the fields, streams and meadows there. He said he found great joy in all the simple things God made—most especially the colorful butterfly, the robin's song, and yes, even the lowly worm. Of course, Brian called the little fellow a "wiggly worm." His love for animals great and small grew out there, out by the meadows and the streams. It was there that he said he felt closest to God.

One morning before Bible study, I found Brian playing his guitar. He said he was writing a new song for the children he was working with—the precious ones that had special challenges. "Please," I asked, "would you share the song with me?" That was many years ago, but I still can remember how my heart was filled with God's joy as Brian sang his new song. Immediately, I began humming and singing along. I couldn't stop laughing—the little song made me *happy!*

The Butterfly Song
by Brian M. Howard

If I were a butterfly,
I'd thank you, Lord, for giving me wings.
If I were a robin in a tree,
I'd thank you, Lord, that I could sing.
If I were a fish in the sea,
I'd wiggle my tail and I'd giggle with glee,
But I just thank you, Father, for making me, *me.*

For you gave me a heart and you gave me a smile,
You gave me Jesus, and you made me your child.
And I just thank you, Father, for making me, me.

If I were an elephant,
I'd thank you, Lord, by raising my trunk.
If I were a kangaroo,
You know I'd hop right up to you.
If I were an octopus,
I'd thank you, Lord, for my fine looks.
But I just thank you, Father, for making me, me.

If I were a wiggly worm,
I'd thank you, Lord, that I could squirm.
If I were a fuzzy, wuzzy bear,
I'd thank you, Lord, for my fuzzy, wuzzy hair.
If I were a crocodile,
I'd thank you, Lord, for my great smile.
But I just thank you, Father, for making me, me.

Brian shared the song at church that day, and everyone, young and old, sang along in no time. Everyone was filled with the same enthusiasm, joy, and childlike wonder that I experienced. In fact, the song became a favorite at our church and we began to sing it regularly. Visitors started sharing it with their own congregations and soon—the song began to travel. We began to hear stories of it traveling all over the country, even the world.

Brian's little song had wings!

The Butterfly Song soon became one of the most popular songs in British schools and churches in Ireland and Scotland.

The song was translated for children in France, Germany, Italy, Spain, Norway, and Sweden. It was sung in Russia and China before flying off to Australia, New Zealand, and South America. Missionaries used the song to teach children of all ages about the love of Jesus and to bring hope to the sick and needy in remote areas around the world.

One day at church, I met Lual (pronounced loo-all), a young man from Africa. He had arrived in America a few days before I met him, and he had never before seen any of the things we associate with modern convenience. He called himself one of the "lost boys" from Southern Sudan, and told me he had learned "The Butterfly Song" in the remote jungle, far away from civilization and long before he had ever seen running water or even a light switch. He had sung the little song with his fellow tribesmen, and it taught him about the love of God.

Over the years, letters and notes have been sent to my friend Brian by children, parents, and grandparents whose lives had been touched in extraordinary ways by singing *The Butterfly Song*. Joyful school children, as well as those who were blind or challenged by other physical disabilities, or those who had suffered child abuse— all were singing the chorus with its simple message of hope.

Numerous publishers recorded the song that earned my friend a certified Gold Record and inclusion on a recording that received a Dove nomination. Orphans in India sang the song on television, and it was broadcast on NBC news. Brian's simple song is often sung at baptisms, graduations, and even funerals. In fact, the song has even been inscribed on a tombstone. *The Butterfly Song,* now a well-known children's classic, continues to be recorded and published worldwide.

The song Brian wrote changed my life and taught me to have a childlike faith. I learned that if God gives us a gift, a talent, or special ability—we must share it. And no talent God gives is small. Songwriting, encouraging, teaching, whatever it is—*share it,* because you just never know what the Lord might do to multiply your gift and then use it to help others.

It was God who gave Brian the meadows and streams, God who made the butterfly that inspired a song beloved the world over and, of course, God who sent Brian to me.

You see, God gave me more than a friendship with Brian. He's still my dearest friend, and I am happy to report that I have been baking him cinnamon rolls for more than 25 years. He is my husband. And I never stop thanking God that I was there with Brian years ago to see the birth of the little song with wings, *The Butterfly Song.*

Your number one magnificent mission is to seek God with all your heart, mind, and soul. God created you to be in fellowship with him every day. Offer your heart and life to God and let him teach you how to live with joy, energy, peace, and purpose. Do the very best you can with what God has given you, and he will use you in ways you can only imagine. He has called you and he will never fail you. It is in God alone that you will find your true fulfillment and the never-ending energy you seek—eternal energy that lasts forever.

> *God doesn't come and go. God lasts.*
> *He's Creator of all you can see or imagine.*
> *He doesn't get tired out, doesn't pause to catch his breath.*
> *And he knows everything, inside and out.*
> *He energizes those who get tired.*
>
> Isaiah 40:28b-29 (MSG)

About the Author

*R*uth Gordon Howard was raised in the Jewish faith. When living in New York City, she had a personal encounter with the living God, and she gave her life to Jesus Christ. As a health care professional and wellness director with over two decades of experience creating health programs for women, she has only one desire—to honor and glorify God in everything she does. She is the creator of the popular program Energy for Working Women® and now Energy for God's Women!™. Ruth is certified by the American College of Sports Medicine and holds a master's degree in health promotion. She is often a radio guest, heard frequently on stations nationwide. She is married to Gold Record award-winning songwriter Brian M. Howard, author of two of the most popular kids' praise songs of all time: *The Butterfly Song (If I Were a Butterfly)* and *I Just Wanna Be a Sheep*.

To correspond with Ruth:
Ruth G. Howard
Energy for God's Women!™
PO Box 470787
Charlotte, NC 28247

For information on booking Ruth for
a speaking engagement:
www.EnergyWomen.com
www.RuthGordonHoward.com
Ruth@EnergyWomen.com
704.442.0620

Visit Brian's & Ruth's music ministry website:
www.ButterflySong.com

Join Us and Be One of the . . .

Energy Girls!®

www.EnergyGirls.com

Join the Energy Girls® Network

If you need more energy,
joy and balance in your life,
if you want inspiration and support,
join our circle of girlfriends and be
one of the Energy Girls®!

Join the Energy Girls® Network and receive :

- News to keep you on track and full of joy.
- Healthy tips and tools that every women needs to be her best.
- Simple, quick, practical help so you can restore the balance in your life.

Get Energy Girls® Info on:

- Having more energy
- Stress management
- Healthy lifestyle tips and tools
- Weight loss
- Organizing your home and work life
- Restoring the balance in your life
- Healing past hurts
- Healthy relationships
- Getting in shape
- Knowing your mission
- Learning how to prioritize
- Simple make ahead meals
- Tips on "Turbo Cleaning"

Sign up online at
www.EnergyGirls.com

Energy
for God's Women!
ENERGY GIRLS® CONTRACT & PLAN

I believe God is calling me to make changes in the following areas:

❏ Use & Discover my Gifts
❏ Develop Godly Relationships
❏ Declutter My Life
❏ Take Care of My Body
❏ Discover and Live My Magnificent Mission

The first change I will make to improve my energy level is . . .

_____

Other changes I will make with God's help . . .

_____

_____

_____

Your Name _____

Date _____

Witness _____

For I can do everything through Christ, who gives me strength.
Philippians 4:13 (NLT)

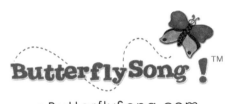

www.ButterflySong.com

The Butterfly Song! CD
If I Were a Butterfly

13 Songs of JOY and TRUTH, including *The Butterfly Song (If I Were a Butterfly)*. All from gold record award-winning songwriter Brian M. Howard. Tons of sing-along fun for the whole family. For Sunday School classes, VBS, Home Schoolers, and families large and small. Includes *The Butterfly Song, He is K-I-N-G, You Come Running*, and *It's a Beautiful Day*.

Price: $14.95 US

Order Online Today!
www.ButterflySong.com

I Just Wanna Be a Sheep CD

12 Songs of JOY and TRUTH, including *I Just Wanna Be a Sheep* and the popular *Armor of God*. You can't help but start singing when you hear these joyous, fun songs! All from gold record award-winning songwriter Brian M. Howard. Tons of sing-along fun for the whole family. For Sunday School classes, VBS, Home Schoolers, and families large and small.

Price: $14.95 US

Order Online Today!
www.ButterflySong.com